Advances in Regional Anesthesia - Future Directions in the Use of Regional Anesthesia

Edited by Eugenio Daniel Martinez Hurtado,
Nekari de Luis Cabezón
and Miguel Ángel Fernández-Vaquero

Published in London, United Kingdom

Advances in Regional Anesthesia - Future Directions in the Use of Regional Anesthesia
http://dx.doi.org/10.5772/intechopen.110961
Edited by Eugenio Daniel Martinez Hurtado, Nekari de Luis Cabezón and Miguel Ángel Fernández-Vaquero

Contributors
Amruta Desai, Ashley Wang, Deborah Li, Eugenio Daniel Martínez Hurtado, Evan Garry, Francisco Fritsch Machry Krum, Freddy Octavio Zambrano Hidalgo, Ian Choe, Javier Aquiles Hidalgo Acosta, Johnny Jerez Castañeda, Juliana María Galán Giraldo, Katrina Kerolus, Kaya Sarier, María Alejandra Morales, María Fernanda Calderón León, Miguel Ángel Fernández Vaquero, Míriam Sánchez Merchante, Nekari de Luis Cabezón, Richard Yeom, Sandra Ximena Jaramillo-Rincón, Sarah Smith, Sergio Bergese, Tiango Aguiar Ribeiro

First published in London, United Kingdom, 2024 by IntechOpen
IntechOpen is the global imprint of INTECHOPEN LIMITED, registered in England and Wales, registration number: 11086078, 5 Princes Gate Court, London, SW7 2QJ, United Kingdom

British Library Cataloguing-in-Publication Data
A catalogue record for this book is available from the British Library

Additional hard and PDF copies can be obtained from orders@intechopen.com

Advances in Regional Anesthesia - Future Directions in the Use of Regional Anesthesia
Edited by Eugenio Daniel Martinez Hurtado, Nekari de Luis Cabezón and Miguel Ángel Fernández-Vaquero
p. cm.
Print ISBN 978-1-83769-350-4
Online ISBN 978-1-83769-349-8
eBook (PDF) ISBN 978-1-83769-351-1

Meet the editors

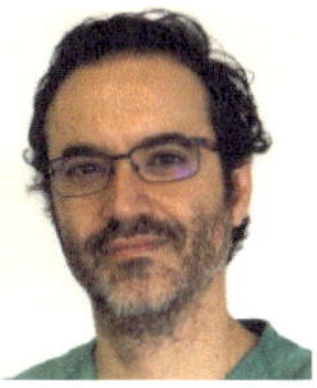

Dr. Martínez Hurtado is a consultant anesthetist, an expert in airway management, and an instructor at the European Airway Management Society (EAMS), Spanish Society of Anesthesiology, Resuscitation and Pain Therapeutics (SEDAR), and Learning, Teaching, and Investigation International Airway Group (FIDIVA). He is also a retired captain of the Spanish Military Health Corps and a teacher of multiple anesthesia and airway management courses at Spanish institutions such as CEU Cardenal Herrera University, University of Alcalá (UAH), and SEDAR PROANES. He has published more than 70 articles in national and international journals and more than 100 conference presentations. Dr. Martínez Hurtado, MD, is a consultant anesthetist in the Department of Anesthesiology and Critical Care Medicine, Infanta Leonor University Hospital, Madrid, Spain. He has master's degrees in anesthesiology, airway management, prevention management (specializing in workplace safety), social and preventive pediatrics, and environmental management. He is a university expert in the fundamentals of community nutrition and a director and professor of international university courses. Dr. Hurtado is an expert in airway management and an instructor certified by the European Airway Management Society (EAMS), Spanish Anesthesia Society (SEDAR), and Investigation International Airway Group (FIDIVA). He is a member of the EAMS Airway Management in Special Circumstances Committee. He is a retired captain of the Spanish Military Health Corps. He is a member of the surgical humanitarian aid campaign at the Hôpital Auberge de l´Amour Rédempteur, Benin, West Africa. He is a journal reviewer and has published more than 70 scientific articles and more than 100 conference presentations.

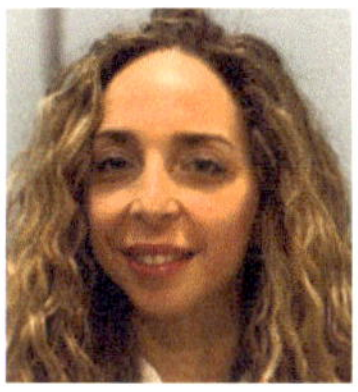

Nekari de Luis Cabezón graduated in medicine from the Vitoria-Gasteiz (UPV-EHU) University of the Basque Country, Spain. She completed her specialization in anesthesiology and resuscitation at the University Hospital of Basurto, Spain in 2013. She completed a university expert training in airway management at the University of Valencia, Spain. She conducted her doctoral thesis on airway point-of-care ultrasound at the Department of Otorhinolaryngology, University of the Basque Country. She is trained by CINEVA/SEDAR as an instructor in difficult airway management. She is also trained as a Teach-the-Airway-Teacher (TaT) by the European Airway Management Society (EAMS). Dr. Cabezón is a professor of various airway courses and workshops, such as the Learning, Teaching, and Investigation International Airway Group (FIDIVA), Difficult Airway Management Workshop, and the European Society of Regional Anaesthesia & Pain Therapy (ESRA) Spain, as well as of airway courses for residents and nursing staff at the University Hospital of Basurto.

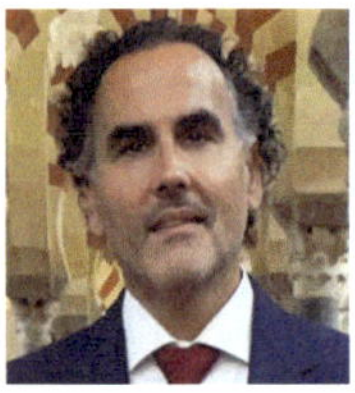

Dr. Miguel Ángel Fernández Vaquero pursued his graduate studies in medicine and surgery at the Faculty of Medicine of Seville from 1994 to 2000. In 2002, he joined the Military Health Corps of the Ministry of Defense of Spain. From 2002 to 2007, he participated in various national and international humanitarian missions with the Spanish Navy. Between 2007 and 2011, he specialized in anesthesiology, intensive care, and pain treatment, completing rotations in significant units in Spain such as the Polytrauma Unit of Albacete University Hospital, the Burn Unit of La Paz University Hospital, and the Cardiac Surgery Unit of Gregorio Marañon University Hospital. In 2011, he was assigned to the Central Defense Hospital in Madrid, Spain. From 2012 to 2018, he undertook international peacekeeping missions with the NATO alliance. From 2013 to 2017, he served as the medical coordinator at the Advanced Pain Management Unit Center at Hospital La Milagrosa. In 2018, he joined the Clinica Universidad de Navarra, where he currently serves as a consultant in the Anesthesiology and Critical Care Department. In 2022, he completed his doctoral thesis on point-of-care ultrasound (PoCUS) for airway management. Dr. Fernández Vaquero is an instructor in Advanced Life Support accredited by the Spanish Society of Intensive and Critical Care Medicine and Coronary Units (SEMYCIUC). Additionally, he teaches PoCUS for Airway Management and Advanced Life Support, Trauma Care, and Airway Management for the Spanish Army. Furthermore, he is a teacher of the International Lung Ultrasound Course alongside Professor Dr. Linchtenstein. Specializing in airway PoCUS, Dr. Fernández Vaquero is recognized as an airway management expert, a European Airway Management Society (EAMS) Airway Management Instructor, and a board member of the Learning, Teaching, and Investigation International Airway Group (FIDIVA). Moreover, he is an instructor for the Teach-the-Airway-Teacher Course with accreditation from the EAMS.

Contents

Preface

Welcome to *Advances in Regional Anesthesia – Future Directions in the Use of Regional Anesthesia*, a comprehensive exploration of the evolving landscape of regional anesthesia. This book provides a cutting-edge perspective on the latest developments, techniques, and research that shape the practice of regional anesthesia today.

Over the years, regional anesthesia has undergone a remarkable transformation, emerging as an integral component of modern perioperative care. As the demand for effective pain management continues to rise, regional anesthesia has proven to be a powerful tool in enhancing patient outcomes, reducing opioid consumption, and improving the overall perioperative experience.

In this volume, we have assembled a distinguished group of experts, clinicians, and researchers who share their insights, experiences, and innovations in the realm of regional anesthesia. The content spans a wide spectrum, from fundamental principles to advanced applications, offering a balanced blend of theory and practical guidance. Readers will find discussions on nerve blocks, catheter techniques, pharmacological advancements, and the integration of technology into regional anesthesia practice.

This book caters to a diverse audience, including anesthesiologists, pain specialists, surgeons, residents, and students interested in the expanding domain of regional anesthesia. Each chapter is crafted to deliver valuable information, foster critical thinking, and inspire further exploration into the ever-evolving field.

The journey through *Advances in Regional Anesthesia – Future Directions in the Use of Regional Anesthesia* takes us beyond traditional boundaries, encouraging practitioners to embrace innovation, evidence-based practice, and collaborative approaches. As we navigate the intricate terrain of regional anesthesia, we are reminded of its pivotal role in achieving optimal patient care and satisfaction.

We extend our sincere gratitude to the contributors who have generously shared their expertise, contributing to the richness and depth of this book. We hope that readers will find this compilation both informative and inspiring, motivating them to embrace and apply the advances presented within these pages.

May this book serve as a valuable resource, fostering a deeper understanding of regional anesthesia and its pivotal role in shaping the future of perioperative medicine.

Eugenio Daniel Martínez Hurtado
Anesthesiology and Resuscitation Service
of Hospital Universitario Infanta Leonor,
Madrid, España

Nekari de Luis Cabezón
Anesthesiology and Resuscitation Service
of Hospital Universitario Basurto,
Bilbao, España

Miguel Ángel Fernández Vaquero
Anesthesiology and Resuscitation Service
of Hospital Clinica Universidad de Navarra,
Madrid, España

Chapter 1

Advances in Regional Obstetric Anesthesia

Francisco Fritsch Machry Krum and Tiango Aguiar Ribeiro

Abstract

Advances in obstetric regional anesthesia, particularly ultrasound-guided techniques, have significantly improved pain relief and safety during childbirth. This chapter explores the latest developments in ultrasound-assisted central neuraxial anesthesia and fascial blocks for post-cesarean analgesia. The use of ultrasound guidance in neuraxial procedures has been extensively studied, demonstrating improved success rates, reduced complications, and increased patient satisfaction. It enhances the accuracy of identifying lumbar intervertebral spaces and facilitates needle insertion, resulting in higher first-pass success rates. Additionally, ultrasound-guided fascial blocks, such as the transversus abdominis plane (TAP) block and Quadratus Lomborum Block (QLB), provide effective analgesia after cesarean section when intrathecal morphine is not feasible. This chapter summarizes the step-by-step technique for ultrasound-guided neuraxial block and fascial blocks, emphasizing the importance of incorporating ultrasound guidance into obstetric anesthesia practice based on the growing body of evidence supporting its benefits.

Keywords: obstetric regional anesthesia, ultrasound-guided, neuraxial block, transversus abdominis block, quadratus lumborum block, post-cesarean analgesia

1. Introduction

Obstetric regional anesthesia has advanced significantly, providing effective pain relief and ensuring the safety of parturients during childbirth. Techniques such as spinal anesthesia and epidural analgesia have revolutionized childbirth care, offering comfort and safety for both mother and baby. With millions of women undergoing childbirth each year, high-quality anesthesia care is crucial for promoting safe deliveries. Technological widespread, including advanced ultrasound techniques, have enhanced precision, safety, and efficacy [1–3]. This chapter explores the latest advancements in ultrasound-assisted central neuraxial anesthesia and fascial blocks for post-cesarean analgesia.

2. Ultrasound-guided neuraxial block

The application of spinal ultrasound for lumbar puncture and neuraxial anesthesia can be attributed to early pioneers such as Bogin, Stulin, Porter, and Cork, who recognized the potential of this technology in locating relevant landmarks [4–6]. Building upon this foundation, subsequent advancements were made by Grau and colleagues, further refining the clinical application of spinal ultrasound and contributing to our current understanding of spinal sonoanatomy [7–9]. Despite notable technical improvements in epidural and spinal procedures, complications such as accidental dural puncture continue to pose concerns. Incorporating ultrasound technology into these procedures holds promise for enhancing safety, improving success rates, and minimizing complications.

In recent years, several systematic reviews and meta-analyses have contributed to the growing body of evidence supporting the use of neuraxial ultrasound. Such reviews demonstrated the superior accuracy of neuraxial ultrasound in identifying lumbar intervertebral spaces compared to landmark palpation alone [10]. Their findings also revealed a strong correlation between ultrasound-measured depth and needle insertion depth, highlighting the precision offered by ultrasound guidance.

Furthermore, it was conducted a review of 32 randomized controlled trials involving 3439 patients in general population. The findings demonstrated that pre-procedural ultrasound not only reduced the failure rate and the need for needle redirections but also increased the first-attempt success rate. Importantly, these improvements were achieved without prolonging the overall procedure time [11].

Similarly, two reviews focusing specifically on the obstetric population, also highlighted the benefits of ultrasound guidance. They found that ultrasound guidance significantly improved the first-pass success rate, with risk ratios of 1.46 (95% CI: 1.16–1.82) and 1.49 (95% CI: 1.21–1.84), respectively [12, 13].

When analyzing the prediction of preprocedural difficulty subgroups, both studies mentioned above also agreed that ultrasound assistance facilitated the first-pass success rate, with risk ratios of 1.56 (95% CI: 1.21–2.01) and 1.40 (95% CI: 1.12–1.75), respectively. Importantly, the use of ultrasound did not increase the total time taken to perform the procedure, with risk ratios of 50.12 (95% CI: −13.69–113.94) and −0.18 (95% CI: −0.86–0.49), respectively [12, 13].

All these studies consistently found a protective association between the use of ultrasound and complications related to the procedure, such as failure of anesthesia, vascular puncture, back pain, and headache. Moreover, one of these studies particularly investigated the differences between the experience of the sonographer and the operator of the procedure. The study found no significant difference between the two groups, especially after considering publication biases [12].

Despite previous descriptions, real-time ultrasound-assisted neuraxial block remains at the forefront of new research studies. Currently, it has been found to be challenging for a single operator to perform and time-consuming compared to the pre-scan technique [14–17]. Furthermore, in anticipation of future advancements in standard care, color Doppler patterns was studied to visualize flow in the epidural space among patients with well-functioning epidural catheters. This pilot study proposes further investigations to identify Doppler patterns in non-functioning catheters to predict the efficacy of this method [18].

These findings collectively emphasize the increasing pool of evidence that supports the use of pre-procedural ultrasound in neuraxial procedures. Aligned with the 2008 recommendation by the National Institute for Health and Care Excellence

(NICE) endorsing the use of ultrasound-guided catheterization of the epidural space, the authors of these studies have unequivocally recommended the incorporation of preprocedural ultrasound in neuraxial procedures [19].

2.1 Technique

The authors summarized the following step-by-step description based on published material from Karmakar, Chin and Carvalho [15, 20]. It should be noted that although being an experienced ultrasound operator does not significantly impact overall success rates, some knowledge of palpation techniques, sonoanatomy, and proficiency with other ultrasound-guided procedures prior to performing neuraxial blocks is expected, considering the delicacy and sensitivity of the region.

Step 1: Begin by communicating the procedure to the patient, ensuring that they understand and provide an opportunity for consent, if applicable. Prepare the ultrasound device by attaching a low frequency curvilinear transducer and adjusting the depth settings to 7 to 10 cm. Organize the necessary devices in a proper arrangement for optimal ergonomics. Perform a thorough equipment safety check, ensuring that all instruments and drugs are appropriately diluted and ready for use.

Step 2: Assisted by another healthcare professional, position the patient in a seated position for the neuraxial procedure, ensuring that the spine is flexed optimally. Put on sterile gloves and thoroughly prepare the skin using an appropriate antiseptic solution. Place a sterile drape over the area and cover the ultrasound transducer with a sterile cap. Apply a generous amount of gel to the transducer to enhance the coupling of ultrasound waves.

Step 3: Palpate the spinous processes to locate the desired area. Instruct the patient to remain as still as possible during the examination and neuraxial anesthesia procedure. We recommend repeating the ultrasound scan and skin markings if the patent moved for any reason.

Step 4: Start your scan 4 to 5 cm lateral to the midline with the transducer longitudinally and, by convention, left side of the screen is cephalad. This will obtain the parasagittal transverse process view where these structures will appear as the "trident sign" pattern. Move transducer medially, 1 to 2 cm lateral to midline to obtain parasagittal articular process view which are seen in a "camel hump" pattern (**Figure 1**).

(Once you have developed proficiency in the sonoanatomy of the region, you can initiate the scan from this point)

Step 5: Gradually move the transducer towards the midline while adjusting the angle of the ultrasound beam by 5 to 10 degrees medially. This will allow you to obtain the parasagittal oblique interlaminar view, as shown in the figure, which displays a distinct "sawtooth" pattern (**Figure 2**). This view provides visualization of the interlaminar spaces as soft gaps. Slide the transducer up and down to identify the optimal interlaminar space for the neuraxial procedure. Once you have identified the optimal view, use a marker to indicate the interlaminar spaces by marking the midpoint of the long edge of the transducer. At this point, use the ultrasound caliper to measure the distance between the skin and the posterior complex. Remember to release the pressure on the transducer when measuring.

Step 6: Rotate the transducer horizontally and medially by 90 degrees to obtain the transverse approach to the spinous process, allowing you to determine the midline. Slide the transducer up or down until you reach the desired interspace. Angling the ultrasound beam by 5 to 10 degrees cephalad will reveal the "bat sign," as shown in the **Figure 3**. The "bat sign" is an important reference for spinal ultrasound as it depicts

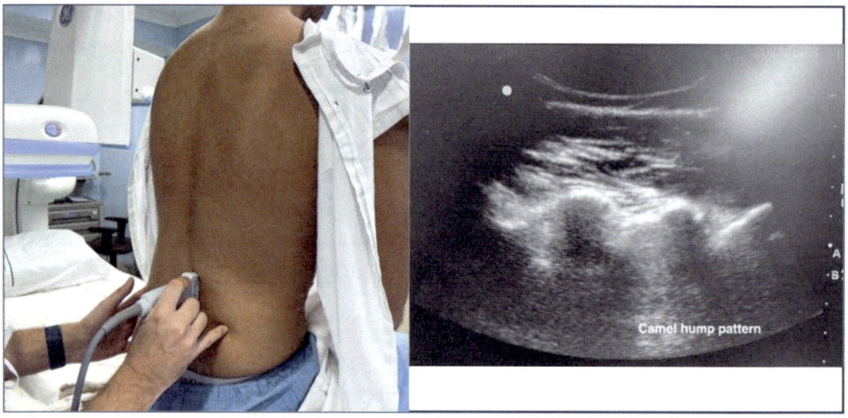

Figure 1.
On the left: Probe positioning. On the right: Camel hump pattern.

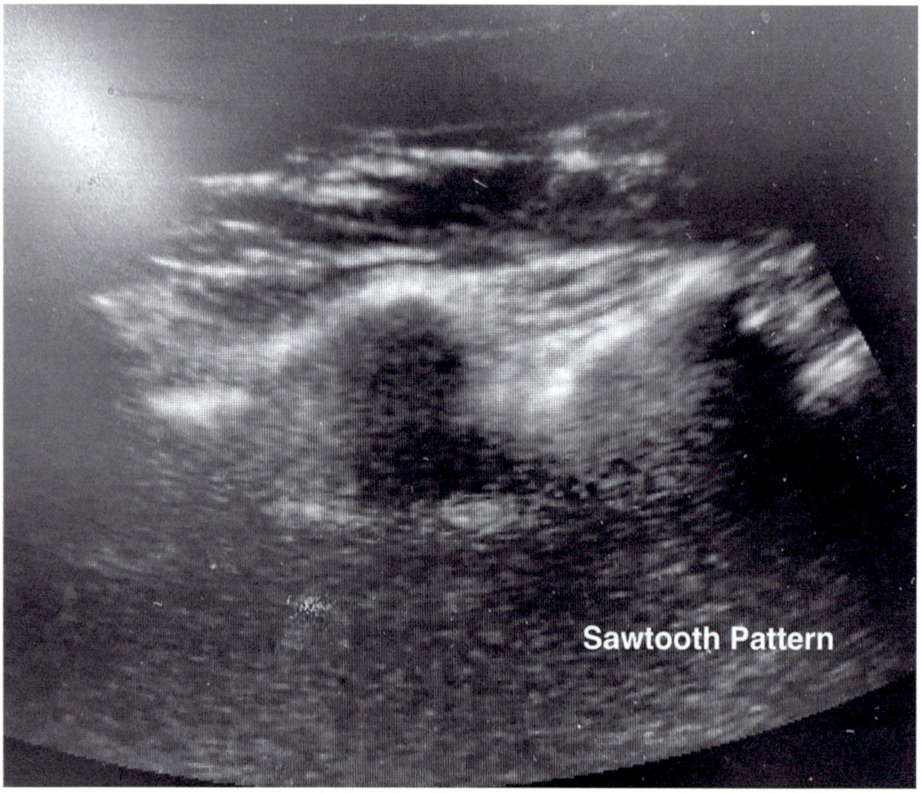

Figure 2.
Sawtooth pattern.

the major anatomical landmarks and targets for neuraxial anesthesia. These include the posterior complex (top of bat's head), anterior complex (bottom of the bat), and the transverse processes (wings of the bat). Select the interspace that provides the clearest view of the "bat sign" to ensure optimal visualization of the posterior and anterior complexes. Align the midpoint of the transducer's long edge with the

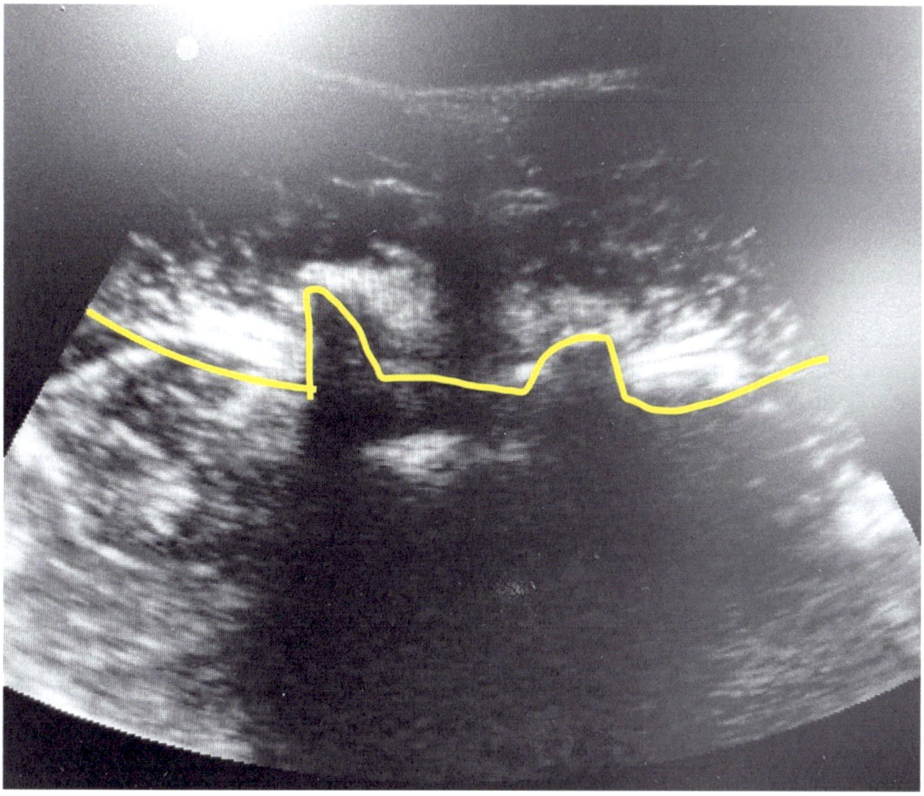

Figure 3.
Bat sign.

patient's midline and use a marker to trace a line that intersects with the horizontal line from the parasagittal view. The crossing of these two lines indicates the site for needle insertion.

Step 7: Use the caliper tool on the ultrasound device to measure the depth of needle insertion from the skin to the posterior complex. Take note of the angle of the ultrasound beam and visually memorize it so that you can replicate this angle during needle insertion.

Step 8: Proceed with the neuraxial procedure following standard practices, using the marked reference points to guide needle insertion and angle. Keep in mind that ultrasound measurements typically underestimate depth by up to 10 mm, with a median underestimation of 3 mm.

3. Ultrasound guided fascial blocks

Cesarean sections often result in moderate-to-severe pain, which can impede recovery, mother-child bonding, and breastfeeding. Multimodal analgesia is crucial for effective postoperative pain management and faster recovery [21]. Intraoperative interventions such as long-acting intrathecal opioids is well known to enhance analgesia after cesarean delivery. But, when such strategy is not feasible, more commonly when spinal anesthesia is contradicted, local analgesia infiltration and abdominal nerve blocks have been found to improve postoperative pain relief [22, 23]. Recommendations by the PROSPECT Working Group [22] and by Enhanced Recovery After Surgery (ERAS) 2019 guideline [23] have guided pain management for cesarean sections with efforts to reduce opioid use and implement enhanced recovery protocols in recent years.

Intrathecal morphine has consistently demonstrated its superiority over fascial blocks for postoperative pain management after cesarean section in various settings, as supported by multiple randomized trials and meta-analyses. High doses of intrathecal morphine have been shown to provide longer-lasting analgesia, albeit with a potential increase in side effects [24–26]. However, in cases where the use of intrathecal morphine is not feasible for cesarean delivery, two fascial blocks can be considered for multimodal analgesia and opioid sparing strategy. These include the Transversus Abdominal Plane Block and Quadratus Lumborum Block. These fascial blocks must be performed bilaterally to cover the cesarean incision and provide adequate analgesia.

There is a limited number of studies directly comparing these techniques with each other. In a 2021 systematic review, despite the low quality evidence, it was found that both TAP Block and QL Block were efficient in reducing pain scores when compared to control groups. Nevertheless, no significant difference was observed between the two techniques in terms of their analgesic efficacy [27]. Further high-quality studies are needed to provide more conclusive evidence on the comparative effectiveness of these fascial blocks for postoperative pain management after cesarean section.

This chapter section will approach each Fascial Block with its rationale and technique. The choice of the technique to use is up to the provider.

3.1 Ultrasound guided transversus abdominal plane block (TAP)

The transversus abdominis plane is a fascial plane located superficially to the transversus abdominis muscle, which is the innermost muscular layer of the anterolateral abdominal wall. The TAP block involves anesthesia of the upper and lower TAP plexuses, formed by the communication of intercostal, subcostal, and L1 segmental nerves.

Since 2021, a group of experts in Regional Anesthesia has worked towards standardizing the terminology for abdominal fascial blocks [28]. One important change is that what was previously known as the Posterior TAP block is now referred to as the Lateral Quadratus Lumborum Block. This standardization requires us to consider the benefits of this approach on the following section of this chapter [29].

As a result of this standardization, Ultrasound-assisted TAP block can be performed using three different approaches: subcostal, transverse abdominal plane, and midaxillary approaches [28]. While each approach has its own specific technique, they all share a common goal of distributing large volumes of local anesthetics within the transverse abdominal plane.

The subcostal approach is believed to provide analgesia for the T6-T9 nerves, while the transverse abdominal plane targets analgesia for the T10-T12 nerves. The midaxillary approach aims to provide analgesia for the lower abdomen, including the L1 nerve. Given our focus on post-cesarean delivery analgesia, we will only describe the midaxillary TAP Block approach.

DOI: http://dx.doi.org/10.5772/intechopen.1002928

3.1.1 Technique

Step 1: Begin by communicating the procedure to the patient, ensuring that they understand and provide an opportunity for consent, if applicable. Prepare the ultrasound device by attaching either a linear or curvilinear transducer and adjusting the depth settings accordingly. Organize the necessary devices in a proper arrangement for optimal ergonomics. Perform a thorough equipment safety check, ensuring that all instruments and drugs are appropriately diluted and ready for use.

TAP blocks are better achieved with high volumes of local anesthetics, with the minimum accepted volume being 15 ml for each side. Select the dosage to achieve the maximum safe dose for the patient's size.

Step 2: TAP Block may be performed by only one provider with the patient on the supine position. Put on sterile gloves and thoroughly prepare the skin using an appropriate antiseptic solution. Place a sterile drape over the area and cover the ultrasound transducer with a sterile cap. Apply a generous amount of gel to the transducer to enhance the coupling of ultrasound waves.

Step 3: Place the transducer transversely on the mid-axillary line of the abdomen and scan the region up and down between the costal margin and the iliac crest. Typically, three muscle layers can be seen: the external and internal obliques, as well as the transverse abdominis muscles (**Figure 4**).

Step 4: Insert the needle in-plane, adjacent to the midaxillary line, and advance it internally and posteriorly. As you advance the needle, you may feel two distinct pops as the needle point passes through the fascia. Once the tip is placed above the TAP, inject the previously selected dosage of local anesthetics, observing the real-time volume spread into the desired space.

Step 5: Repeat the process on the other side.

3.2 Ultrasound guided quadratus Lumborum block

The quadratus lumborum (QL) is a muscle of the posterior abdominal wall dorsolateral to the psoas major muscle. Originating from the iliac crest and iliolumbar

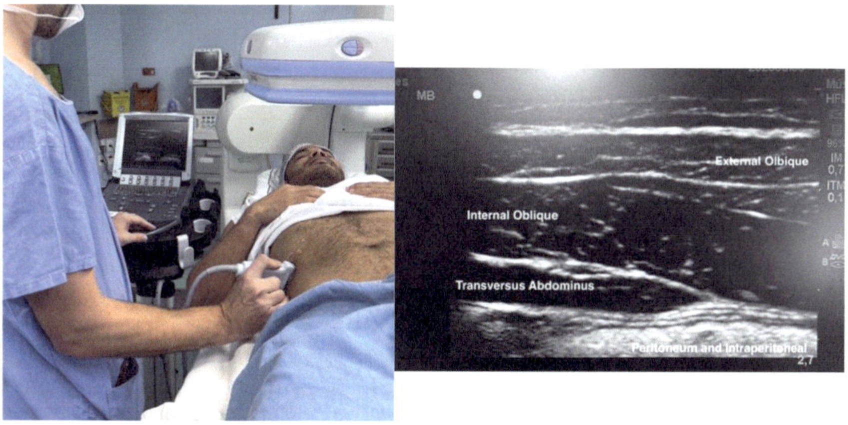

Figure 4.
On the left: Probe positioning. On the right: Sonoanatomy of the region.

ligament, the QL muscle assists in lateral flexion of the lumbar spine. The QL block has gained popularity in different abdominal surgeries as a tool for multimodal analgesia because of its theoretical efficiency over visceral pain [30].

In a 2020 meta-analysis, which reviewed 12 studies involving 904 patients undergoing cesarean delivery, quadratus lumborum block (QLB) was found to significantly reduce opioid (intravenous morphine) consumption during the first 24 hours by 14.1 mg (95% CI 20.8 to 7.5 mg) and 48 hours by 20.8 mg (95% CI 33.1 to 8.5 mg) compared to placebo or no block. Additionally, QLB demonstrated a significant reduction in 12-hour pain scores at rest and during movement [30].

Similarly, QLB reduced opioid consumption compared to controls and provided better pain control at 6 and 12 hours postoperatively. While no significant differences in pain scores were noted at 24 hours, QLB was effective in reducing dynamic pain at 6 hours and both static pain and opioid consumption at 6 and 12 hours [31].

The terminology for QL Blocks, similar to TAP Blocks, has been standardized by a group of experts in Regional Anesthesia [28]. This standardization has led to the recognition of three possible approaches for achieving adequate analgesia: Anterior Quadratus Lumborum Block, Lateral Quadratus Lumborum Block, and Posterior Quadratus Lumborum Block [32, 33]. However, clinical studies directly comparing these three methods are lacking, and only cadaveric studies have suggested variations in the spread of local anesthetics with each approach [33].

Given that the Posterior Quadratus Lumborum Block is the most extensively studied approach for providing analgesia after cesarean delivery [34, 35], we will now review its step-by-step technique.

3.2.1 Technique

Step 1: Begin by communicating the procedure to the patient, ensuring that they understand and provide an opportunity for consent, if applicable. Prepare the ultrasound device by attaching preferably low frequency curvilinear transducer and adjusting the depth settings accordingly. Organize the necessary devices in a proper arrangement for optimal ergonomics. Perform a thorough equipment safety check, ensuring that all instruments and drugs are appropriately diluted and ready for use.

Local anesthetic dosage in the range of 0.2 to 0.4 ml/kg of 0.2 to 0.5% ropivacaine or 0.1 to 0.25% bupivacaine per side is recommended. The operator will need to adjust dosage to ensure toxic thresholds are not exceeded, particularly when bilateral blocks are performed.

Step 2: QL Block may be performed by only one provider with the patient on lateral decubitus or supine with a lateral tilt. Put on sterile gloves and thoroughly prepare the skin using an appropriate antiseptic solution. Place a sterile drape over the area and cover the ultrasound transducer with a sterile cap. Apply a generous amount of gel to the transducer to enhance the coupling of ultrasound waves.

Step 3: Place the transducer transversely on the posterior axillary line of the abdomen at the L4 level. Visualize the "shamrock sign" where the transverse process serves as the stem, and the psoas, quadratus lumborum, and erector spinae muscles form the leaves. Utilize color Doppler to ensure safe needle trajectory, avoiding any large vessels along the way (**Figure 5**).

Step 4: Insert the needle in-plane and advance it internally and posteriorly. Position the needle tip posterior to the QL muscle within the fascia adjacent to the erector spinae muscle. To confirm proper needle tip placement, inject 2 ml of saline

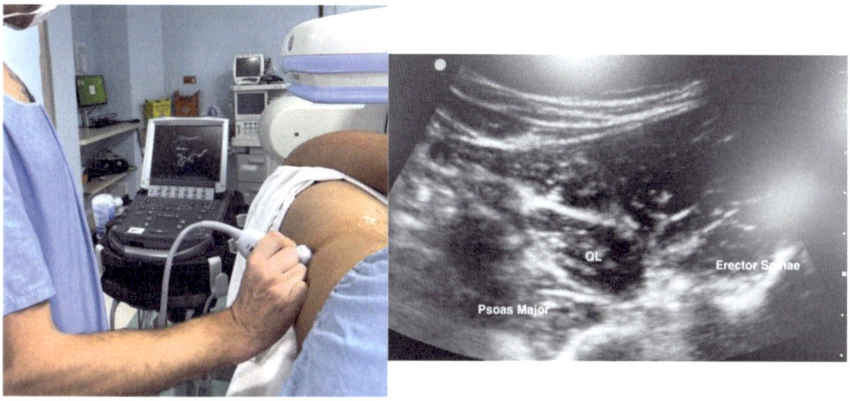

Figure 5.
On the left: Probe positioning. On the right sonoanatomy of the region.

before administering the total dose. Monitor the spread of local anesthetic as you inject slowly.

Step 5: Repeat the process on the other side.

4. Conclusion

Anesthesia care, over the past two decades, has integrated the use of ultrasound-guided procedures. The combination of professional expertise with the use of ultrasound guidance, can further elevate the level of care and ensure the well-being of their patients. As we look to the future, the continuous evolution of ultrasound technology and its increasing availability hold the promise of even greater advancements in safety, comfort, and positive outcomes for patients globally.

Author details

Francisco Fritsch Machry Krum and Tiango Aguiar Ribeiro*
Program of Health Science, Federal University of Santa Maria (UFSM), Santa Maria, Rio Grande do Sul, Brazil

*Address all correspondence to: tiangoribeiro@gmail.com

References

[1] Aveline C. Regional anesthesia in obstetrics: Where are we now? Current Opinion in Anesthesiology. 2017;**30**(3):289-293. DOI: 10.1097/ACO.0000000000000450

[2] Wong C. Advances in regional anesthesia for labor and delivery. Regional Anesthesia and Pain Medicine. 2017;**42**(3):251-259. DOI: 10.1097/AAP.0000000000000599

[3] Reynolds F. Obstetric anaesthesia and analgesia. Anaesthesia. 2015;**70**:95-109. DOI: 10.1111/anae.12859

[4] Bogin I, Stulin I. Application of the method of 2-dimensional echospondylography for determining landmarks in lumbar punctures. Zhurnal Nevropatologii i Psikhiatrii Imeni S.S. Korsakova. 1971;**71**:1810-1811

[5] Porter R, Wicks M, Ottewell D. Measurement of the spinal canal by diagnostic ultrasound. Journal of Bone and Joint Surgery - British. 1978;**60**:481-484

[6] Cork R, Kryc J, Vaughan R. Ultrasonic localization of the lumbar epidural space. Anesthesiology. 1980;**52**:513-516

[7] Grau T, Leipold R, Horter J, Conradi R, Martin E, Motsch J. Paramedian access to the epidural space: The optimum window for ultrasound imaging. Journal of Clinical Anesthesia. 2001;**13**:213-217

[8] Grau T, Bartusseck E, Conradi R, Martin E, Motsch J. Ultrasound imaging improves learning curves in obstetric epidural anesthesia: A preliminary study. Canadian Journal of Anaesthesia. 2003;**50**:1047-1050

[9] Grau T. The evaluation of ultrasound imaging for neuraxial anesthesia. Canadian Journal of Anaesthesia. 2003;**50**:R1-R8

[10] Perlas A, Chaparro L, Chin K. Lumbar Neuraxial ultrasound for spinal and epidural Anesthesia: A systematic review and meta-analysis. Regional Anesthesia and Pain Medicine. 2016;**41**(2):251-260. DOI: 10.1097/AAP.0000000000000184

[11] Sidiropoulou T, Christodoulaki K, Siristatidis C. Pre-procedural lumbar Neuraxial ultrasound—A systematic review of randomized controlled trials and meta-analysis. Healthcare. 2021;**9**:479. DOI: 10.3390/healthcare9040479

[12] Young B, Onwochei D, Desai N. Conventional landmark palpation vs. preprocedural ultrasound for neuraxial analgesia and anaesthesia in obstetrics - a systematic review and meta-analysis with trial sequential analyses. Anaesthesia. 2021;**76**(6):818-831. DOI: 10.1111/anae.15255

[13] Jiang L, Zhang F, Wei N, Lv J, Chen W, Dai Z. Could preprocedural ultrasound increase the first-pass success rate of neuraxial anesthesia in obstetrics? A systematic review and meta-analysis of randomized controlled trials. Journal of Anesthesia. 2020;**34**(3):434-444. DOI: 10.1007/s00540-020-02750-6

[14] Grau T, Leipold R, Fatehi S, Martin E, Motsch J. Real-time ultrasonic observation of combined spinal-epidural anaesthesia. European Academy of Anaesthesiology. 2004;**21**(1):25-31. DOI: 10.1017/s026502150400105x

[15] Karmakar M, Chin K. Spinal sonography and applications of

ultrasound for central neuraxial blocks [Internet]. 2017. Available from: https://www.nysora.com/techniques/neuraxial-and-perineuraxial-techniques/spinal-sonography-and-applications-of-ultrasound-for-central-neuraxial-blocks [Access at: 2023-04-18]

[16] Conroy P, Luyet C, McCartney C, McHardy P. Real-time ultrasound-guided spinal anaesthesia: A prospective observational study of a new approach. Anesthesiology Research and Practice. 2013;**2013**:525818. DOI: 10.1155/2013/525818

[17] Chen L, Huang J, Zhang Y, Qu B, Wu X, Ma W, et al. Real-time ultrasound-guided versus ultrasound-assisted spinal Anesthesia in elderly patients with hip fractures: A randomized controlled trial. Anesthesia and Analgesia. 2022;**134**(2):400-409. DOI: 10.1213/ANE.0000000000005778

[18] Van den Bosch O, Gleicher Y, Arzola C, Siddiqui N, Downey K, Carvalho J. Color flow Doppler in spinal ultrasound: A novel technique for assessment of catheter position in labor epidurals. Regional Anesthesia and Pain Medicine. 2022;**47**(12):775-779. DOI: 10.1136/rapm-2022-103948

[19] National Institute for Health and Care Excellence. Ultrasound guided catheterisation of the epidural space: understanding. IPG249. 2008

[20] Carvalho J. Ultrasound-facilitated epidurals and spinals in obstetrics. Anesthesiology Clinics. 2008;**26**(1):145-158. DOI: 10.1016/j.anclin.2007.11.007

[21] Ciechanowicz S, Setty T, Robson E, Sathasivam C, Chazapis M, Dick J, et al. Development and evaluation of an obstetric quality-of-recovery score (ObsQoR-11) after elective caesarean delivery. British Journal of Anaesthesia. 2019;**122**(1):69-78. DOI: 10.1016/j.bja.2018.06.011

[22] Roofthooft E, Joshi G, Rawal N, Van de Velde M. PROSPECT working group* of the European Society of Regional Anaesthesia and Pain Therapy and supported by the obstetric anaesthetists' association. PROSPECT guideline for elective caesarean section: Updated systematic review and procedure-specific postoperative pain management recommendations. Anaesthesia. 2021;**76**(5):665-680. DOI: 10.1111/anae.15339

[23] Macones GA, Caughey AB, Wood SL, Wrench IJ, Huang J, Norman M, et al. Guidelines for postoperative care in cesarean delivery: Enhanced recovery after surgery (ERAS) society recommendations (part 3). American Journal of Obstetrics and Gynecology. 2019;**221**(3):221-247. DOI: 10.1016/j.ajog.2019.04.012

[24] Fusco P, Scimia P, Paladini G. Transversus abdominis plane block for analgesia after Cesarean delivery. A systematic review. Minerva Anestesiologica. 2015;**81**:195-204

[25] Champaneria R, Shah L, Wilson M, Daniels J. Clinical effectiveness of transversus abdominis plane (TAP) blocks for pain relief after caesarean section: A meta-analysis. International Journal of Obstetric Anesthesia. 2016;**28**:45-60

[26] Ng S, Habib A, Sodha S, Carvalho B, Sultan P. High-dose versus low-dose local anaesthetic for transversus abdominis plane block post-caesarean delivery analgesia: A meta- analysis. British Journal of Anaesthesia. 2018;**120**:252-263

[27] El-Boghdadly K, Desai N, Halpern S, Blake L, Odor PM, Bampoe S, et al. Quadratus lumborum block vs.

transversus abdominis plane block for caesarean delivery: A systematic review and network meta-analysis. Anaesthesia. 2021;**76**(3):393-403. DOI: 10.1111/anae.15160

[28] El-Boghdadly K, Wolmarans M, Stengel AD, et al. Standardizing nomenclature in regional anesthesia: An ASRA-ESRA Delphi consensus study of abdominal wall, paraspinal, and chest wall blocks. Regional Anesthesia & Pain Medicine. 2021;**46**:571-580. DOI: 10.1136/rapm-2020-102451

[29] Faiz S, Alebouyeh M, Derakhshan P, Imani F, Rahimzadeh P, Ashtiani M. Comparison of ultrasound-guided posterior transversus abdominis plane block and lateral transversus plane block for postoperative pain management in patients undergoing caesarean section: A randomized double-blind clinical trial. Journal of Pain Research. 2017;**11**:5-9

[30] Xu M, Tang Y, Wang J, Yang J. Quadratus lumborum block for postoperative analgesia after cesarean delivery: A systematic review and meta-analysis. International Journal of Obstetric Anesthesia. 2020;**42**:87-98. DOI: 10.1016/j.ijoa.2020.02.005

[31] Tsai H, Yoshida T, Chuang T, Yang S, Chang C, Yao H, et al. Transversus abdominis plane block: An updated review of anatomy and techniques. BioMed Research International. 2017;**2017**:8284363. DOI: 10.1155/2017/8284363

[32] Ueshima H, Otake H, Lin JA. Ultrasound-guided quadratus lumborum block: An updated review of anatomy and techniques. BioMed Research International. 2017;**2017**:2752876. DOI: 10.1155/2017/2752876

[33] Elsharkawy H, El-Boghdadly K, Barrington M. Quadratus Lumborum block: Anatomical concepts, mechanisms, and techniques. Anesthesiology. 2019;**130**(2):322-335. DOI: 10.1097/ALN.0000000000002524

[34] Blanco R, Ansari T, Girgis E. Quadratus lumborum block for postoperative pain after caesarean section: A randomised controlled trial. European Journal of Anaesthesiology. 2015;**32**:812-818

[35] Blanco R, Ansari T, Riad W, Shetty N. Quadratus lumborum block versus transversus abdominis plane block for postoperative pain after cesarean delivery: A randomized controlled trial. Regional Anesthesia and Pain Medicine. 2016;**41**:757-762

Chapter 2

PoCUS and Regional Anesthesia for Airway Management

Eugenio Daniel Martínez Hurtado,
Nekari de Luis Cabezón, Miguel Ángel Fernández Vaquero
and Míriam Sánchez Merchante

Abstract

Point-of-care ultrasound (PoCUS) has emerged as a valuable tool in regional anesthesia and airway management. The chapter begins with an overview of PoCUS and its relevance to anesthetic practice, highlighting its advantages and limitations, and emphasizing the potential benefits of PoCUS in improving the accuracy and safety of regional anesthesia procedures, leading to enhanced patient outcomes. Furthermore, the chapter explores the utility of PoCUS in airway management, including the assessment of the upper airway, identification of anatomical locations, and real-time visualization of needle placement during airway blocks. Additionally, the chapter addresses the practical aspects of incorporating PoCUS into the daily practice of anesthesiologists, including the necessary equipment, technique considerations, and training requirements. It emphasizes the importance of proper education and ongoing proficiency in PoCUS to optimize its clinical utility and ensure accurate interpretation of images, optimizing patient care. Overall, this book chapter provides a comprehensive overview of the integration of PoCUS with regional anesthesia techniques and airway management, serving as a valuable resource for anesthesiologists, trainees, and allied healthcare professionals interested in enhancing their knowledge and skills.

Keywords: point-of-care ultrasound, PoCUS, regional anesthesia, airway management, healthcare, learning, patient care

1. Introduction

Up to 30% of adverse effects solely attributed to the anesthesia procedure are related to the airway pathway. The majority of these are due to the inability of orotracheal intubation (or errors in it) or difficulty in ventilation. The consequences are catastrophic, and although the more widespread use of capnography and pulse oximetry has reduced these adverse effects, patients can still experience irreversible brain damage or death in up to 85% of cases [1–4].

Therefore, proper management of the airway constitutes one of the fundamental pillars of medical care in certain specialties (anesthesiology, intensive care, emergency medicine, or pulmonology). However, an inadequate approach still represents one of the leading causes of morbidity and mortality among patients, as well as demands in these specialty fields.

In order to approach an airway and to anticipate and manage both foreseeable and unexpected difficulties, different strategies need to be developed, starting with patient assessment, including medical history and specific physical examination.

When predictors suggest a difficult airway (DA) (either due to previous surgeries or highly indicative DA prediction tests), prioritizing oxygenation and ventilation while causing minimal damage to the airway pathway is crucial. In cases where DA is anticipated, the safest and standard technique is considered to be vigil intubation [5]. However, this approach to the airway pathway induces greater physical and psychological stress for the operator, which can lead to suboptimal execution of the technique, a higher number of complications, and even procedure failure. Moreover, certain patient characteristics such as obesity, prior cervical radiotherapy, presence of masses, and cervical scars or abscesses can hinder its proper execution.

With the patient awake, any airway device can be used, as long as proper preparation with local anesthesia and sedation is performed. Regional anesthesia (RA) of the airway pathway provides adequate anesthesia of all its structures, allowing intubation to be performed without sedation or with minimal doses, with very good tolerance and patient cooperation with spontaneous ventilation and preserved reflexes. Similarly, it can be useful in patients where we want to reduce the autonomic response to endotracheal intubation and minimize the doses of drugs used in anesthesia induction [6].

2. Basic aspects

For awake intubation, there is no single method to approach the procedure. Different strategies of premedication, sedation, and topicalization can be employed to maintain a level of patient consciousness that ensures proper airway and spontaneous ventilation, with adequate anxiolysis to tolerate the procedure [7].

All physicians responsible for managing an advanced airway device (DA) should be trained in performing awake intubation. Whether through nasal or oral route, tracheostomy, or cricothyrotomy, awake intubation allows for maintaining airway patency, gas exchange, and protection against aspiration of gastric contents or blood.

The most common technique is performing awake intubation using a fiberoptic bronchoscope (FOB) or videoendoscope, but it can also be done with other devices such as videolaryngoscopes (VDL), optical stylets, lighted stylets, or supraglottic devices, which are used to pass the FOB through them [8–14].

The preferred technique for intubation in these cases remains the use of FOB, although there are increasing studies suggesting videolaryngoscopy as an alternative, with the patient awake or, if not feasible, in spontaneous ventilation (in case the patient refuses the awake procedure) [15]. Supporting the procedure with an inhalation induction technique and topical anesthesia of the airway can enhance its effectiveness [16].

3. Anatomy

The upper airway is divided into four zones encompassing a total of five nerves, which provide sensory innervation to the airway (**Figures 1** and **2**, **Table 1**):

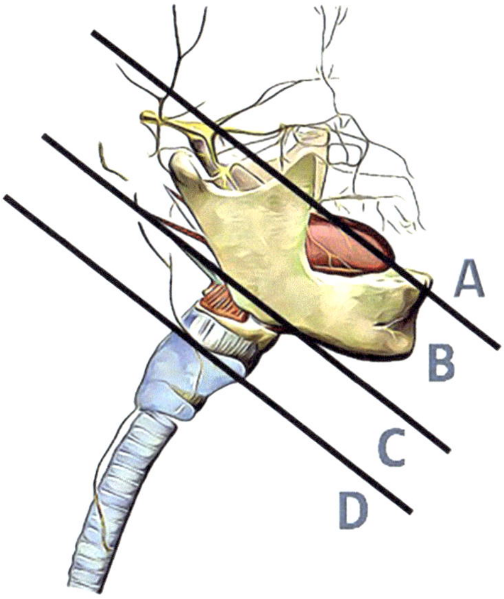

Figure 1.
The upper airway sensory innervation division, by Fernandez-Vaquero [17].

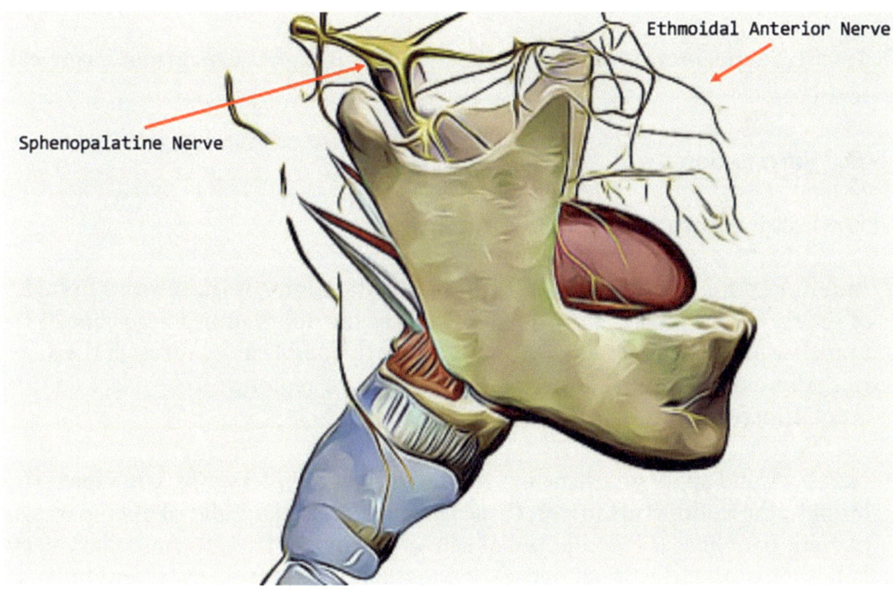

Figure 2.
Nasal innervation, by Fernandez-Vaquero [17].

A. Nasal zone, innervated by the trigeminal nerve (anterior ethmoidal and maxillary/sphenopalatine branches).

B. Oral zone, innervated by the glossopharyngeal nerve.

Zone	Nerve	Branches and areas
Nasopharynx	Branches of the Trigeminal nerve (V cranial nerve)	• Ophthalmic branch: anterior ethmoidal nerve. • Nasal cavity: anterior 1/3 of nostrils. • Maxillary branch: nasal cavity: nasal turbinates and posterior 2/3 of nasal septum.
Oropharynx	Glossopharyngeal nerve (IX cranial nerve)	• Posterior 1/3 of tongue, anterior surface of epiglottis and vallecula (lingual branch), tonsils (tonsillar branch), pharyngeal walls, and tonsillar pillars (pharyngeal branch). • Nausea reflex.
Larynx	Vagus nerve (X cranial nerve)	• Superior laryngeal nerve: base of tongue, posterior area of epiglottis, aryepiglottic folds, and arytenoids. • Recurrent laryngeal nerve: vocal cords and infraglottic region.
Trachea	Vagus nerve (X cranial nerve)	• Recurrent laryngeal nerve: Abduction of vocal cords. Sensation in the infraglottic larynx and trachea.

Table 1.
Innervation of different regions of the airway. Nerve branches and areas.

C. Laryngeal zone, innervated by the vagus nerve through its superior laryngeal and recurrent branches.

D. Tracheal zone, innervated by the vagus nerve through the recurrent laryngeal branches.

3.1 Nasal innervation

It is primarily provided by two branches:

- Anterior ethmoidal nerve. Located in the orbital cavity, is the sensory branch of the nasociliary nerve and, also, a branch of the ophthalmic nerve (one of the branches of the trigeminal [V PC]). It enters the nasal cavity through the anterior ethmoidal foramen. It innervates the anterior region and the nasal septum. It is not directly accessible for blocking (**Figure 2**).

- Maxillary and sphenopalatine nerves. Located in the pterygopalatine fossa (posterior to the middle turbinate), these nerves form a triangular-shaped parasympathetic ganglion. It is composed of sensory branches from the maxillary nerve (a branch of the trigeminal nerve), sympathetic fibers from the carotid plexus (after reaching the ganglion through the vidian nerve, a branch of the greater petrosal nerve), and parasympathetic fibers from the communicating branches of the glossopharyngeal nerve. From it emerge the greater and lesser palatine nerves, which supply sensory innervation to the nasal cavity (nasal passages and posterior two-thirds of the nasal septum), the roof of the mouth, the soft palate, and the tonsils. Other important branches of the maxillary nerve that innervate the nasal cavity are the posterosuperior lateral and inferoposterior branches (**Figure 2**).

3.2 Innervation of the oropharyngeal zone is determined by the glossopharyngeal nerve

- Glossopharyngeal nerve. A mixed nerve supplies sensory innervation to the posterior third of the tongue (gag reflex and the sense of taste), pharyngeal walls (pharyngeal branch), tonsils (tonsillar branch), and the anterior surface of the epiglottis (lingual branch) (**Table 1**).

3.3 Innervation of the laryngeal zone is determined by the vagus nerve through two of its branches

- Superior laryngeal nerve (**Table 1**). It runs parallel to the superior thyroid vessels (branches of the external carotid artery), descends anterior to it to the greater horn of the hyoid bone, dividing into a mainly motor external branch (which innervates the cricothyroid and inferior pharyngeal constrictor muscle), and a sensitive internal branch (which innervates the base of the tongue, the epiglottis and the supraglottic mucosa of the larynx). The level of division into its terminal branches varies greatly. Its injury causes dysphonia.

  The superior laryngeal nerve provides sensory innervation (internal branch) and motor innervation to the supraglottic portion of the larynx: cricothyroid muscle and the inferior constrictor of the pharynx. The level at which it divides into its internal and external terminal branches varies greatly.

- Recurrent laryngeal nerve. It supplies sensory innervation to the infraglottic region and trachea and motor innervation by the external branch of the superior laryngeal nerve (except to the cricothyroid muscle, which is innervated by the external branch of the superior laryngeal nerve). It runs parallel to the inferior thyroid artery. Its injury causes inability to abduct the vocal cords (closed vocal cords) and secondary airway obstruction (**Table 1**).

3.4 Innervation of the tracheal zone is determined by the vagus nerve through its recurrent laryngeal branch

4. Practical considerations

ALR for performing awake intubation, whether orotracheal or nasotracheal, can be carried out using the following methods:

4.1 Topicalization with local anesthetic (LA)

There are different forms of application [18]:

4.1.1 Nebulization (8–10 mL of 5% lidocaine with an oxygen flow of 8 L)

The respiratory tract can be anesthetized with lidocaine through a nebulizer. Particles larger than 100 μm will concentrate in the oral mucosa, those between 60 and 100 μm in the trachea and main bronchi, and those between 60 and 30 μm. in the larger bronchi. In the nebulizer, 8–10 mL of 5% lidocaine is placed, and oxygen is released with an 8 L/min flow.

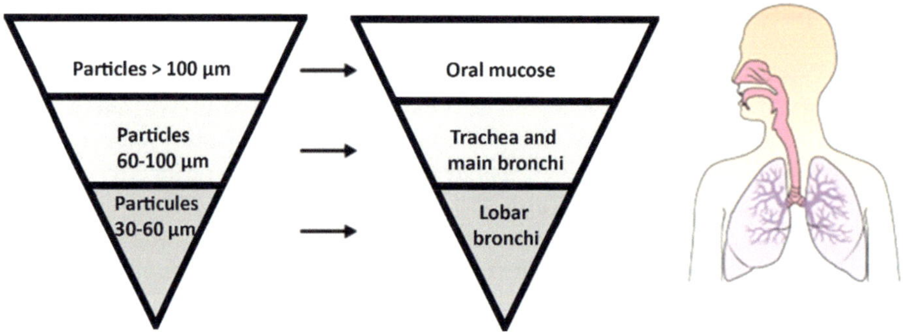

Figure 3.
Airway nebulization, by Fernandez-Vaquero [17].

This is an easy, safe, non-invasive, and comfortable technique for the patient. Coughing is minimal or absent. It requires 20 to 30 minutes to achieve adequate anesthesia. Absorption varies; therefore, high doses are sometimes used to compensate for this limitation (**Figure 3**).

4.1.2 Direct application of lidocaine gel or spray

Currently, the atomizer spray (MADgic atomizer) is used, as it is the most effective, easiest to apply, and most commonly used. With gauze or swabs. This method is useful for applying lidocaine with vasoconstrictor in the nasal cavity. When performing nasal intubation, it is important to prepare the nasal mucosa with a vasoconstrictor to minimize the risk of bleeding. A rhinoscope and special otolaryngology forceps are used to introduce the swabs soaked with the anesthetic into the back of the nasal cavity (5% lidocaine with 0.5 mL. of oxymetazoline, 4% lidocaine with adrenaline 1,200,000 as the vasoconstrictor or 10 mg./ml. tetracaine with 0.1 mg./ml. epinephrine). The local anesthetic should be deposited in the space behind the inferior turbinate along the floor of the nose to the choana. This anesthetizes the nose and part of the oropharynx as the anesthetic falls by gravity toward these structures.

4.1.3 "Spray as you go" (SAYGo)

It consists of applying local anesthetic through the working channel of the Fiber-Optic Bronchoscope (FOB) to the mucosa of the airways as it is advanced.

If a small syringe is used for application, the local anesthetic may stay in the channel instead of reaching the mucous membrane of the respiratory tract. To prevent this, 2 mL. of 5% lidocaine is loaded into a 10 mL. syringe and the remaining space is filled with air. This creates a mixture of lidocaine and air. In this way, a greater force is created when the plunger is pressed, and the lidocaine falls to the distal part of the working channel almost like a jet.

The local anesthetic can also be instilled through an epidural catheter placed in the working channel. Normally, this maneuver should be performed by an assistant. It may cause coughing. If the anesthetic is introduced with less force, the risk of coughing is reduced. When the spray falls, the FOB's vision will become blurry. It is necessary to administer O2 or ask the patient to take a deep breath to regain clear vision.

4.2 Regional nerve blocks providing sensation to the airways in their three regions

Blocks can be performed by locating anatomical structures or by using ultrasound, with the latter technique offering greater safety by avoiding accidental puncture of blood vessels or other structures adjacent to the airway, such as the thyroid gland. Additionally, it allows for the identification of structures even in patients with more complex anatomy (obese patients, previous surgeries, goiter, etc.) [19]. Ultrasound has become an essential tool in the daily practice of every physician, especially in anesthesiology, as it greatly enhances patient safety throughout the perioperative period, whether by performing nerve blocks, vascular access, intraoperative ultrasound for hemodynamic management, or any other use that improves the quality of care. It is a technique that offers many obvious advantages (safety, speed, repeatability, portability, wide availability, and real-time dynamic imaging). It has been demonstrated that even in expert hands, only three out of every 10 specialists are capable of locating the cricothyroid membrane based solely on anatomical references [6]. Tracheal structures can be identified by ultrasound, even when they are not palpable [20, 21].

Ultrasound of the airway has a steep learning curve and is operator-dependent, although basic structure identification can be acquired with just a few hours of training. For this purpose, a high-frequency linear probe (5–14 MHz.) is probably the most suitable since it deals with superficial structures (within 0–5 cm. below the skin surface) [22].

Regional blocks, ideally guided by ultrasound, are indicated in cases where topical anesthesia is contraindicated or not recommended, has been ineffective, or when the depth of the nerve prevents topical blockade. They involve the injection of a local anesthetic into the territory of a nerve to produce anesthesia in the area [19, 23–25].

Specific nerve blocks can be performed for the following nerves:

- Palatine nerve (sphenopalatine ganglion)
- Glossopharyngeal nerve
- Superior laryngeal nerve
- Inferior or recurrent laryngeal nerve

Regional/topical anesthesia of the airway provides adequate anesthesia of all its structures and allows for intubation (orotracheal or nasotracheal) without sedation or with minimal doses, with very good patient tolerance and cooperation, spontaneous ventilation, and preserved reflexes. In addition to patient tolerance, it can be useful to inhibit reflex responses provoked by intubation, such as coughing or laryngospasm [26, 27], as well as sympathetic nervous system-mediated cardiovascular responses [23, 28].

5. Applied anatomy for anesthetic management of the airway

Practically speaking, we will divide the innervation of the airway into the four previously mentioned zones: nasal, innervated by the trigeminal nerve; oral-pharyngeal, innervated by the glossopharyngeal nerve; laryngeal, innervated by the vagus nerve through its superior and recurrent laryngeal branches; and tracheal, innervated by the vagus nerve through its recurrent laryngeal branch.

5.1 Nasal zone

For this zone, topical anesthesia is commonly used due to its high efficacy and good patient tolerance, the high risk of vascular puncture in palatine nerve blocks, and the inaccessibility of the anterior ethmoidal nerve.

5.1.1 Topical anesthesia

By direct contact with swabs or pledgets (4 mL. of 5% lidocaine with 0.5 mL. of 0.5% oxymetazoline or 4% lidocaine with 1,200,000 adrenaline) on the posterior space behind the inferior turbinate (identified using a rhinoscope) (**Figure 4**).

5.1.2 Sphenopalatine ganglion block

Blockade of the sphenopalatine ganglion, by blocking the greater and lesser palatine nerves, the nasociliary nerve, and the nasopalatine nerves, inhibits the sensitivity of the nasal cavity. Two approaches have been described: intraoral and nasal [19].

In order to visualize the blockage point of the greater palatine nerve and to perform the intraoral approach, the patient is placed in the supine position with a pillow under the shoulders, with the mouth open and the chin elevated (**Figure 5**). With the operator to the right of the patient, the right hand is placed at the 8 o'clock position and the left hand at 4 o'clock. The greater palatine foramen is identified with the aid of a swab, usually (in 50% of cases) 1 cm medial to the space between the second and third molars, or slightly anterior (39%) or posterior. At that level, pressure is applied with the swab on the palatogingival border until the depression caused by the foramen is felt.

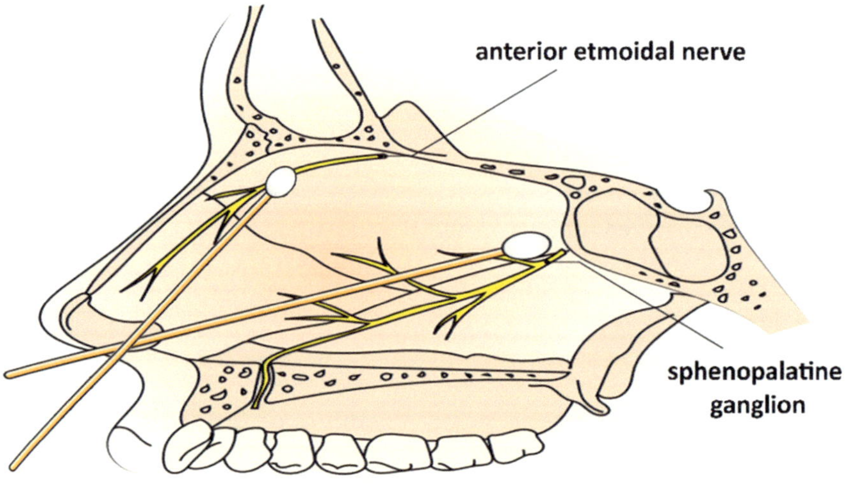

Figure 4.
Direct contact block of the sphenopalatine and anterior ethmoid nerves, by Fernandez-Vaquero [17].

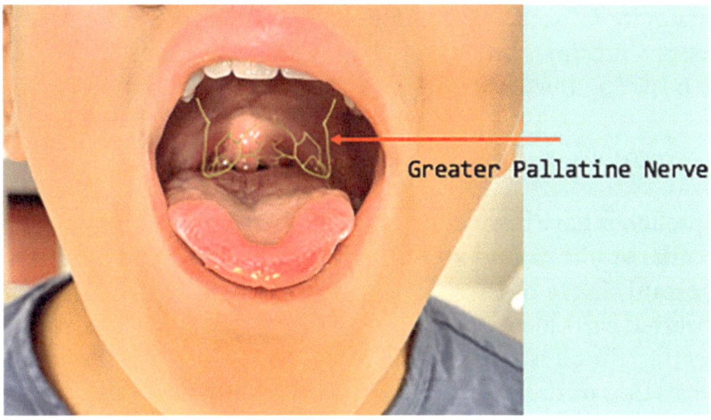

Figure 5.
Intraoral major palatine nerve blockage, by Fernandez-Vaquero [17].

Once the foramen is located, a fine needle (25G or 27G spinal needle bent at approximately 120° about 2–3 cm. from the tip) is inserted 1–2 mm. anterior to the foramen, in a superior direction with a slight posterior inclination until bone contact is felt. Prior to aspiration in two planes (the original plane and rotating the needle 45°), 1–2 mL. of local anesthetic (2% lidocaine with 1,100,000 adrenaline) is injected at a very slow speed (approximately 1 minute) to avoid sympathetic stimulation. In 5–15% of cases, resistance may be encountered when inserting the needle into the canal, at which point the technique should be stopped and alternatives sought.

Complications include hemorrhage, infection, nerve injury, and intravascular injection of local anesthetic.

This technique is contraindicated in cases of acute inflammatory or infectious processes in the puncture area.

On the other hand, in the nasal approach to perform the nasopalatine nerve block, the anesthetic solution is applied with swabs on the upper edge of the middle turbinate (3 mL. of 4–5% lidocaine with 1 mL. of oxymetazoline). The swab shall be introduced at a 45° angle to the hard palate, directed posteriorly and inferiorly until it reaches the posterior wall of the nasopharynx. It can also be performed using a 20G catheter in the same location.

5.2 Oropharyngeal zone

The responsible nerve for the sensory innervation of the oropharynx is the glossopharyngeal nerve. Topical anesthesia is usually sufficient for upper airway instrumentation, although it must be accompanied by preventive measures for nausea and vomiting as it does not reach the receptors of the posterior third of the tongue. Glossopharyngeal nerve blockade, however, does inhibit the gag reflex as it is able to block the deep sensitivity of the posterior third of the tongue, so bilateral gag reflex blockade is used to abolish it.

5.2.1 Topical anesthesia

Topical anesthesia of the glossopharyngeal nerve is performed using swabs or cotton swabs. Swabs soaked in 5% lidocaine (mixed with 10 mL. of 5% lidocaine solution) are used. It is inserted into the channel between the teeth and the tongue until it reaches the palatoglossal arch. The swab is held in place for approximately 1 minute, repeating three or four times on each side. Always check that the topicalization is correct before inserting the device.

5.2.2 Glossopharyngeal block

Several approaches have been described using visualization and palpation of anatomical landmarks or ultrasound guidance (the latter being the preferred method). The most important risk to be taken into account is vascular puncture due to the proximity of the internal carotid artery and jugular vein, which will be avoided by aspirating before injecting the anesthetic [19]. Given the proximity to the carotid artery and jugular vein, injection of the anesthetic should be stopped in case of headache.

5.2.2.1 Glossopharyngeal block using anatomical landmarks

- Intraoral or anterior approach (palatoglossal or anterior pillar). With the patient seated with the mouth open, the block is approached from the opposite side of the target nerve. Once appropriate topical anesthesia (lidocaine spray) has been administered, the tongue is pulled toward the midline using a laryngoscope blade or tongue depressor, while directing the 22-25G needle along the floor of the mouth down to the bottom of the pouch formed by the base of the palatoglossal arch. Once negative aspiration is confirmed, 2–5 mL. of 2% lidocaine is injected into the submucosa (**Figure 6**).

- Posterior intraoral approach (palatopharyngeal or posterior tonsillar pillar). With the patient seated, the nerve is approached from the same side as the blockage by puncturing the palatopharyngeal cavity approximately 0.5 cm. lateral to the lateral edge of the tongue, where it joins the floor of the mouth, at the base of the posterior tonsillar pillar, blocking both the sensory and motor branches. A 22-23G needle is inserted up to 1 cm., and after aspiration, 3 mL. of 0.5–1% lidocaine (with a test dose of 0.5 mL.) are injected slowly, following verification

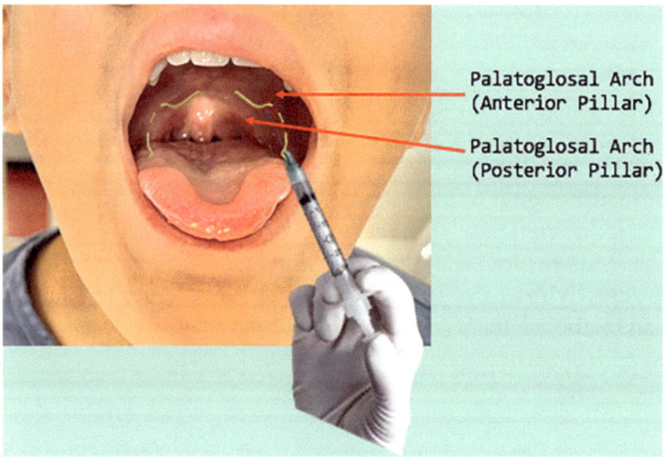

Figure 6.
Blockage of the glossopharyngeal nerve at the level of the palatoglossal archs, by Fernandez-Vaquero [17].

through aspiration. Alternatively, an anesthetic-soaked pledget can be applied to the area to be blocked instead of puncture.

The injection is bilateral, blocking the sensory fibers (pharyngeal, lingual, and tonsillar) and the motor branch of the stylopharyngeus muscle, with a consequent increased risk of complications.

- Peristyloid external approach. This approach is indicated when the patient cannot open their mouth wide enough to adequately expose the structures. The mastoid process and the angle of the mandible shall be located by placing the patient in the supine position with the head in a neutral position. The styloid process (next to the glossopharyngeal nerve, which runs adjacent to the internal carotid artery) is located by deep palpation or at the midpoint of the line drawn from the mastoid process to the mandibular angle. At this point, a 22G needle is inserted perpendicular to the skin until it comes into contact with the bone (1–2 cm), then angled to inject 5–7 mL of the anesthetic solution (2% lidocaine) after verification by aspiration. Peristyloid approach guided by ultrasound is recommended.

5.2.2.2 Ultrasound-guided glossopharyngeal nerve block

With the patient in the supine position and the head tilted to the contralateral side of the block, the cervical region shall be scanned with a high-frequency linear ultrasound transducer or a hockey stick probe to locate the mastoid process, mandibular angle, and styloid process at the midpoint, usually with the probe in an oblique transverse axis. At this point, the vessels (carotid artery and jugular vein) are identified using Doppler ultrasound, and the glossopharyngeal nerve is identified as a hyperechoic structure posterior and deeper to the styloid process and anterior to the carotid artery (**Figure 7**).

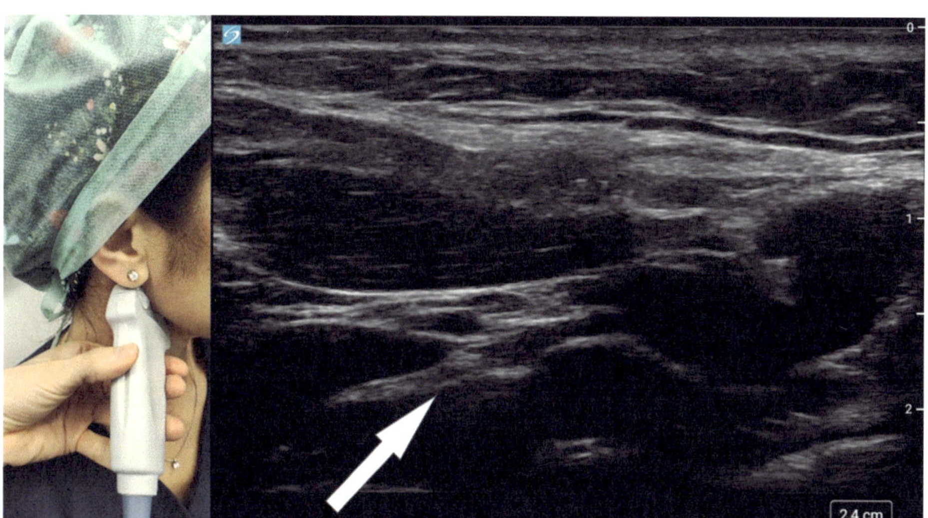

Figure 7.
Glossopharyngeal nerve block by ultrasound-guided peristylohyoid approach. The transducer is placed between the mandibular angle and the mastoid process and angled to locate the styloid process, carotid artery, and external jugular vein. The glossopharyngeal nerve is located posterior to the styloid process, by Fernandez-Vaquero [17].

The puncture is performed out of the plane until contacting the styloid process, and then the needle is redirected posteriorly to inject 3 mL of local anesthetic after aspiration to ensure that there is no blood or cerebrospinal fluid leakage.

Proper alignment of the transducer is crucial in Doppler effect usage: ideally, it should be positioned parallel to the blood flow (if not possible, at an angle of 0–60°). The Doppler effect can be enhanced by increasing the ultrasound frequency, increasing the flow velocity, or decreasing the transducer angle relative to the vessel or structure to be visualized.

Conventionally, blue represents the flow moving away from the transducer (longer wavelengths), and red represents the flow moving toward the transducer (shorter wavelengths).

5.3 Laryngeal region

5.3.1 Topical anesthesia

The larynx is innervated by branches of the vagus nerve (superior and recurrent laryngeal nerves). To anesthetize the supraglottic laryngeal region, topical anesthesia shall be applied in the piriform recess. This procedure requires proper oral opening, time, and prior preparation of the oropharynx, which is why it is infrequently used. If this is insufficient, the blockage of the superior laryngeal nerve can be performed, although it is less commonly used and has a higher number of complications (vascular injection, severe vagal reactions, etc.). The vocal cords are not completely paralyzed.

5.3.2 Superior laryngeal nerve block

Bilateral blockade of the superior laryngeal nerve results in anesthesia of the hypopharynx and upper glottis, including the vallecula and the posterior surface of the epiglottis. The main indication for this blockage is to facilitate the management of a difficult airway associated with local anesthetic nebulization in the oral/nasal and transtracheal cavities. Its blockage inhibits the gag reflex and coughing provides supraglottic anesthesia and minimizes the risk of laryngospasm by preventing the contraction of the cricothyroid muscle. It has been used in awake fiberoptic intubation and rigid bronchoscopy procedures (**Table 2**) [29, 30].

Other indications include as an alternative to neuromuscular blockers in case of contraindication (myasthenia gravis, dystrophies, etc.) and the treatment of persistent headaches due to superior laryngeal nerve neuralgia [31]. Classically, it is located by palpation. With the patient in the supine position and the head extended and tilted laterally to the side opposite to the block, locate the greater horn of the hyoid bone or the thyroid cartilage (upper horn or midline prominence) [19].

	Topical anesthesia	**Nerve block**
Control of secretions	Atropine required	Not required
Anesthetic dose	10 mg./spray lidocaine 10%.	Lower dose (2 mL.)
Blocking duration	Lower	Longer
Need for repeat doses	More frequent	No

Table 2.
Comparison between topical anesthesia and upper laryngeal blockade.

A 25G needle is then inserted perpendicular to the plane of the skin to a depth of 1–2 cm until the bone is palpated, at which point it is redirected anteroinferiorly toward the midline to penetrate the thyrohyoid membrane at a depth of 2–3 mm. Using the superior horn of the thyroid cartilage as a reference, in this case, after inserting the needle and hitting the cartilage, it is angled anterosuperiorly to locate the thyrohyoid membrane, where a loss of resistance is felt (**Figure 8**).

Another possibility is to palpate the thyroid notch, puncturing at a suprathyroid level 2 cm. from the midline, and directing the needle cranially and posteriorly until the thyroid membrane is located at a depth of 1–2 cm.

Before injecting the anesthetic (2 mL. of 2% lidocaine with 1/200,000 adrenaline), negative aspiration should be checked (neither air, indicating excessive depth, nor blood should appear).

The use of ultrasound is recommended for the localization of the hyoid bone and the cricothyroid membrane (**Figure 9**), as the technique is safer with a lower risk of complications, such as vascular puncture, among others [32].

Ideally, a hockey stick transducer is used, which provides higher resolution and smaller size, allowing for more maneuverability of the needle. However, a linear or convex probe is typically used. The in-plane approach is recommended to control the needle tip due to the limited space available and to avoid injury to adjacent structures.

Different approaches can be considered:

- Barberet's approach: a high-frequency linear transducer is placed in a parasagittal axis at the submandibular level. The hyoid bone, the upper edge of the thyroid cartilage, the muscles of the vocal cords (omohyoid, sternohyoid, and thyrohyoid), the artery, and the superior laryngeal nerve (between the muscles and the thyrohyoid membrane) are identified, as well as the internal laryngeal mucosa. The cartilage and bone are hyperechoic structures, among which the thyrohyoid

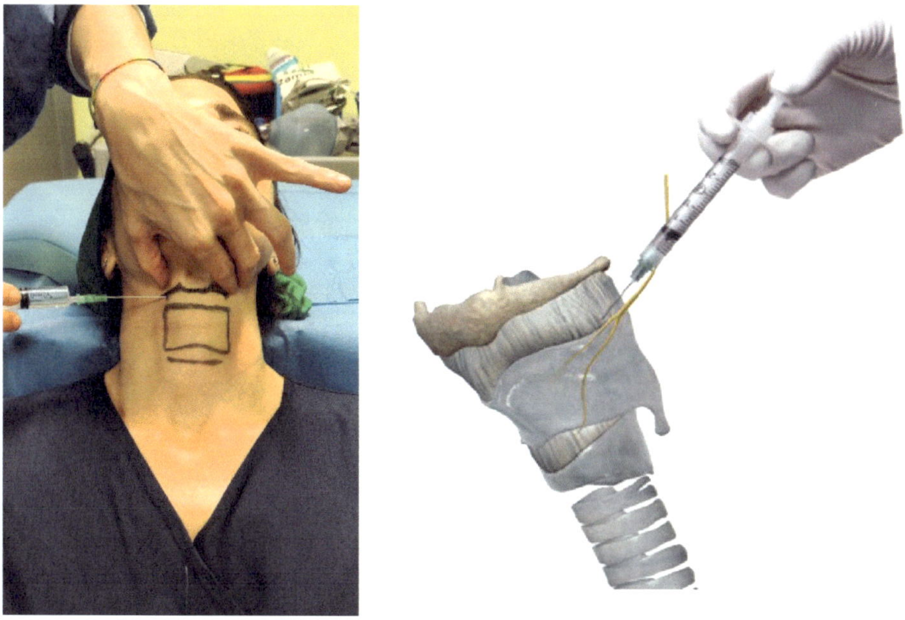

Figure 8.
Superior laryngeal nerve block guided by anatomical references, by Fernandez-Vaquero [17].

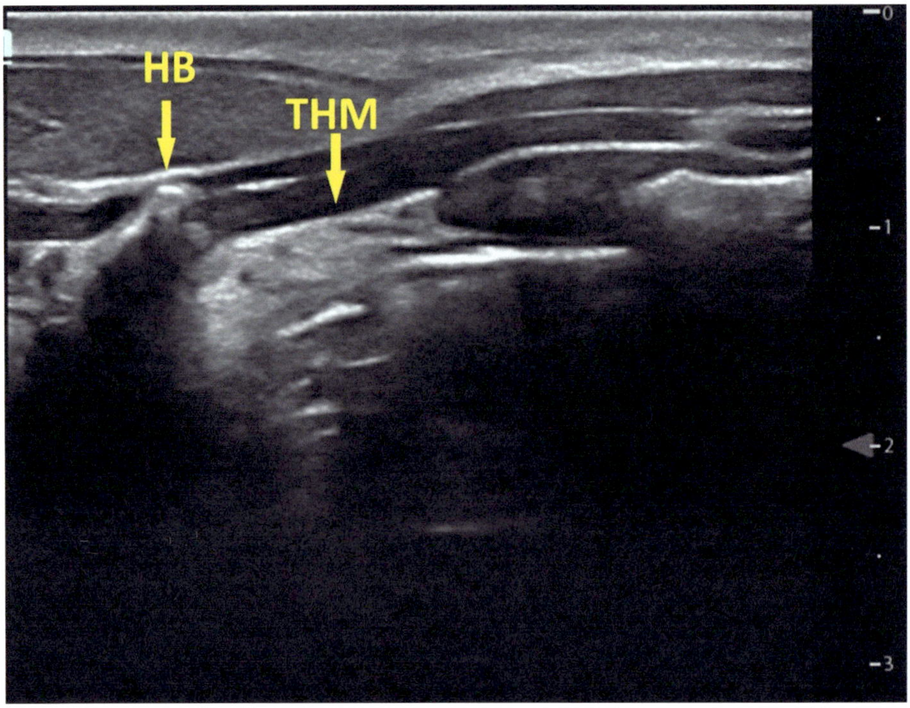

Figure 9.
HB: Hyoid bone; THM: Thyrohyoid membrane, by Fernandez-Vaquero [17].

membrane is located. At this level, local anesthetic is bilaterally injected. This technique has a success rate of 90% [33].

- Manikandan's approach: the submandibular region is explored to locate the external carotid artery and, following its branches, to visualize the superior laryngeal nerve [25].

- Lida's approach: the greater horn of the hyoid bone is identified without visualizing the superior laryngeal nerve [24].

- Transverse axis approach with a probe, in case of technical impossibility or contraindication for the longitudinal approach or non-visualization of the nerve (<1 mm. diameter) [34].

An attempt should be made to avoid the potential risk of broncho-aspiration: it is necessary to observe the required fasting time, maintain an appropriate level of consciousness, and adopt an anti-Trendelenburg position upon awakening. The duration of supraglottic anesthesia will depend on the anesthetic used. The blockage of the superior laryngeal nerve should be complemented with topical anesthesia of the nasal and oral cavities, as well as transtracheal nebulization. The external branch of the superior laryngeal nerve can be injured during neck surgeries.

There are various degrees of injury, although clinically it is characterized by a slight deterioration in voice quality. Anesthesia of the superior laryngeal nerve can cause Wallerian degeneration with damage to the Schwann cell and axonal dystrophy, characterized by mild hoarseness. The use of a linear probe requires greater pressure on the neck, resulting in pain.

5.4 Tracheal zone

5.4.1 Blockage of the recurrent laryngeal nerve

The recurrent laryngeal nerve is a mixed nerve with intrinsically connected motor and sensory fibers. Blocking it would cause bilateral paralysis of the vocal cords and obstruction of the airway, so it is contraindicated.

However, it is necessary to block it to prevent coughing and allow the passage of the tracheal tube or fibroscope through the vocal cords. For this purpose, topical anesthesia of the mucosa is advised, using the "as you go" technique or through transtracheal or translaryngeal blockage.

5.4.2 Translaryngeal or transtracheal blockage

The patient is placed in a supine position with the neck extended (ideally with a pillow under the shoulders), which makes the laryngeal structures more prominent.

The classic approach is blindly performed by palpating the cricoid cartilage in the midline. The larynx is stabilized with the first and second fingers of one hand; after identifying the upper edge of the cartilage, a subcutaneous wheal is formed with the free hand, and a 20-22G needle is inserted perpendicularly to the skin until it traverses the cricothyroid membrane, which is confirmed by the continuous aspiration of air (bubbling). At that moment, the needle is secured to prevent puncturing the posterior wall, and 5 mL. of 4% lidocaine are rapidly injected. The injection of the anesthetic stimulates coughing, which nebulizes the anesthetic and blocks the recurrent laryngeal nerve (**Figure 10**). After the procedure, the needle is quickly withdrawn, and a catheter can be left in place if further doses are anticipated to prolong the blockade.

Ultrasound-guided approach facilitates the localization of the cricothyroid membrane between the thyroid and cricoid cartilages, as well as the control of needle tip placement into the laryngeal lumen, ensuring proper deposition of the anesthetic through translaryngeal blockade. Among the advantages of the ultrasound-guided approach are the more precise localization of blood vessels (avoiding the risk of bleeding and VA hematomas) and the possibility of confirming the correct placement of the tracheal tube [24, 32].

Caudocranial scanning of the neck allows differentiation of the tracheal cartilage, the cricoid cartilage, and the thyroid cartilage. The cricothyroid membrane is echogenic (white), although it may vary in appearance depending on the anatomy, and is located between the caudal edge of the thyroid cartilage (hypoechogenic or gray) and the cephalic boundary of the cricoid cartilage (hypoechogenic or gray) and the cricothyroid muscles. Ultrasound waves do not penetrate air, therefore the posterior wall of the larynx cannot be visualized.

Ultrasound Guided Approach Cricothyroid Membrane Localization:

- Position: patient in supine position.

- Probe: linear, depth 3–4 cm., and focus at 1 cm.

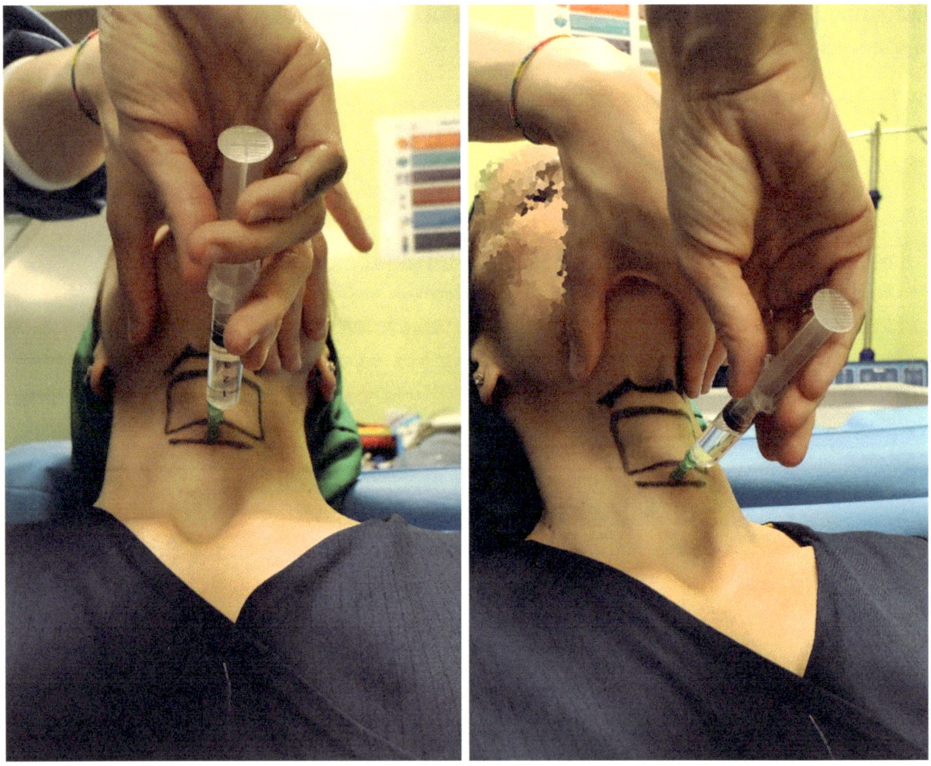

Figure 10.
Translaryngeal block through the cricothyroid membrane using anatomical landmarks, by Fernandez-Vaquero [17].

Exploration Procedure:

Transverse Section:

1. Thyroid cartilage level: a triangular structure with a delta wing shape is observed. The vocal cords will appear inside with a triangular shape. (Requires angulation of the probe at 45–60° in a cephalic direction).

2. Cricoid cartilage level: for the second cut, slide the probe caudally until the next semicircular cartilaginous structure, which is the cricoid cartilage.

3. Tracheal rings level: for the third transverse cut, direct the probe caudally until it reaches the tracheal rings. At the level of the 6th or 7th tracheal ring, stop the probe and rotate it 90° on its own axis, thus achieving the change from transverse to longitudinal exploration.

Longitudinal Section:

4. Cricoid cartilage and tracheal rings: hypoechoic images in the form of "lentils" (tracheal rings) and a larger, rounder structure in a cephalic position resembling a "bean" (cricoid cartilage) are observed.

DOI: http://dx.doi.org/10.5772/intechopen.1003842

5. Thyroid-cricoid cartilage (cricothyroid membrane): in a cephalic direction, once the cricoid cartilage is identified, the tissue that appears just after it is the cricothyroid membrane, which inserts in a cephalic position on the thyroid cartilage (**Figure 11**).

Cricothyroid Membrane Marking:

1. Preparation of marking kit and needle placement: a Tuohy needle or another guide needle can be used, along with a vial of methylene blue for coloring. Position the needle between the skin and probe, creating a hyperechoic image on the superficial part with subsequent acoustic shadowing. Then, move it to the upper edge of the cricoid cartilage.

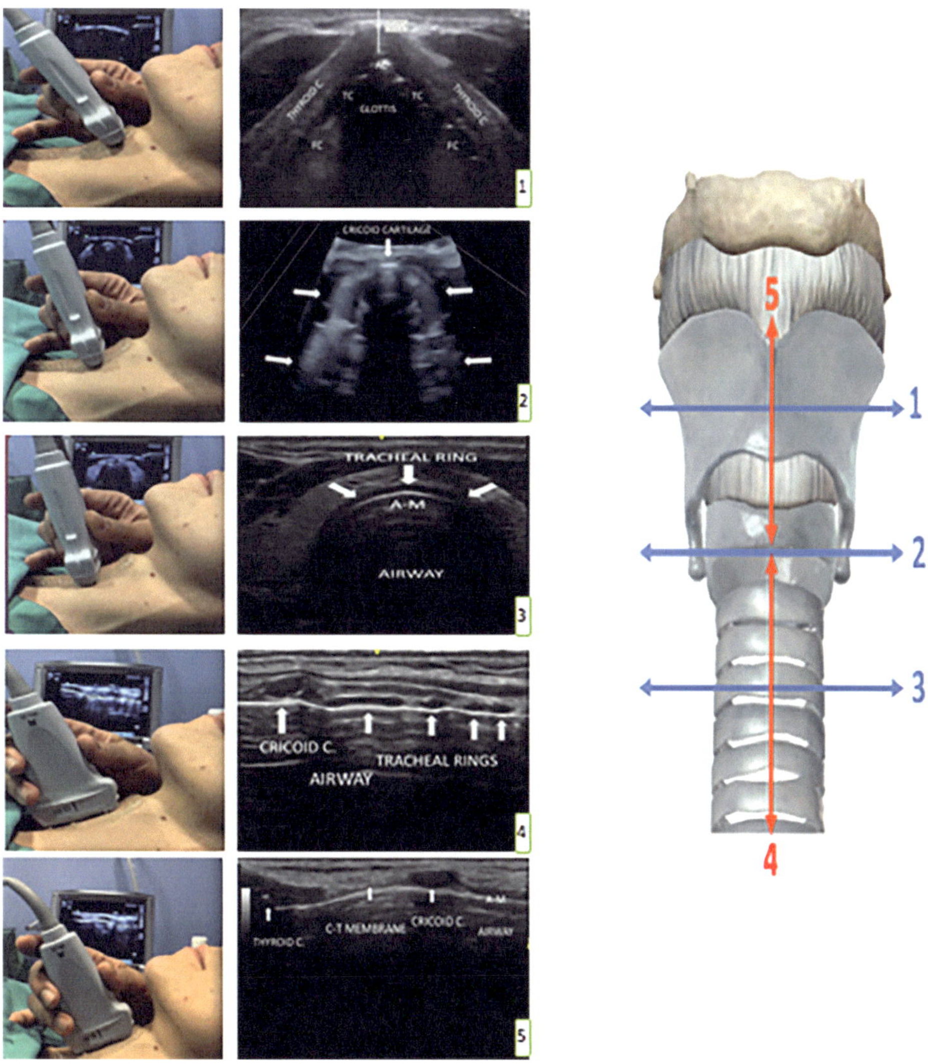

Figure 11.
Ultrasound-guided approach for the localization of the cricothyroid membrane, by Fernandez-Vaquero [17].

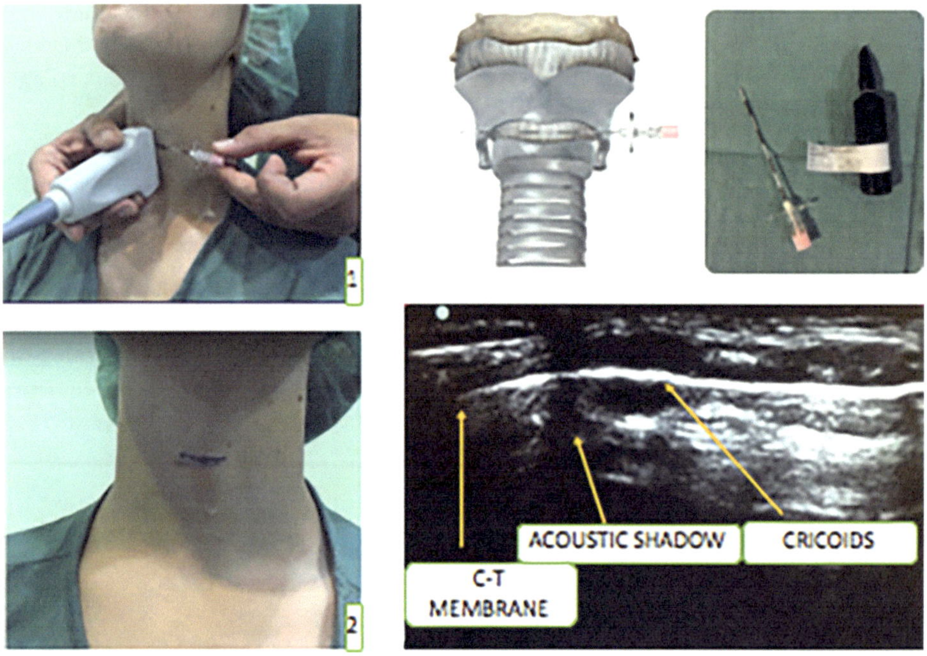

Figure 12.
Cricothyroid membrane marking, by Fernandez-Vaquero [17].

2. Membrane marking: finally, upon needle removal, a mark will remain at the level of the lower border of the cricothyroid membrane. If measurements of the membrane have been taken, a millimeter ruler can be used to draw the entire thickness (**Figure 12**).

Maintaining the probe with the membrane in the center of the image, the exact location is marked with a pen or needle, or a subcutaneous wheal is created and the prelaryngeal space is measured to calculate the maximum needle insertion length, which is inserted in a caudal direction on a plane. Once air aspiration is confirmed, 4 mL of 2% lidocaine is injected. Ultrasound localization surpasses palpation and surface anatomical references (usual maneuver) in terms of time and effectiveness. Additionally, it allows for confirmation of the tracheal tube placement and identification of potential procedure-related complications.

Real-time visualization of laryngeal vessels is also facilitated. It is important not to lose sight of the superior and inferior laryngeal vessels or the needle tip. Since intralaryngeal air hinders visibility of the needle's posterior part, it is recommended to measure the anteroposterior laryngeal diameter and clamp the needle to a length smaller than this diameter to prevent perforation of the vessels, mediastinitis, and/or laryngoesophageal fistula [35].

The following complications of translaryngeal block can occur: bleeding, infection, and tracheal perforation (secondary pneumomediastinum, subcutaneous emphysema, and esophageal perforation). This block should not be performed in patients at risk of aspiration, coagulation disorders, or cervical instability.

6. Conclusions

- The main indication for regional anesthesia of the laryngeal vestibule (LV) is awake intubation in difficult airways. There is no single approach for the total LV block.
- The most commonly used technique is topical anesthesia or direct application of local anesthetic (LA) to the LV. The least invasive technique should be chosen, with a preference for topical anesthesia over nerve blocks.
- To select an appropriate regional anesthesia, it is crucial to individualize the technique based on the objectives, characteristics of the procedure, patient, and environment. Likewise, a comprehensive knowledge of the anatomy and physical principles of ultrasound equipment is essential.
- The use of ultrasound is recommended to enhance the safety and efficiency of anesthesia, as well as to combine necessary blocks. Ultrasound minimizes complications, but in-depth anatomical knowledge of the blocking area is indispensable.
- Regional techniques complement oxygenation, adequate sedation, and anti-emetic measures, with proper patient information. Among the most commonly used techniques are anesthetic topicalization and blocks of the glossopharyngeal, superior laryngeal, and translaryngeal nerves.
- Any instrumentation of the LV can cause trauma or adverse effects such as edema, hemorrhage, esophageal or tracheal perforation, pneumothorax, or bronchoaspiration.
- Pediatric patients, polytraumatized patients, patients with full stomach or glottic/subglottic obstruction, and obstetric patients require special treatment.

Conflict of interest

The authors declare no conflict of interest.
All images are original works of the authors.

Author details

Eugenio Daniel Martínez Hurtado[1]*, Nekari de Luis Cabezón[2], Miguel Ángel Fernández Vaquero[3] and Míriam Sánchez Merchante[4]

1 Infanta Leonor University Hospital, Madrid, Spain

2 Basurto University Hospital, Bilbao, Spain,

3 University of Navarra Clinic, Madrid, Spain,

4 Alcorcón Foundation University Hospital, Madrid, Spain

*Address all correspondence to: eugeniodaniel.martinez@salud.madrid.org

References

[1] Caplan RA, Posner KL, Ward RJ, Cheney FW. Adverse respiratory events in anesthesia: A closed claims analysis. Anesthesiology. 1990;**72**(5):828-833

[2] Cheney FW, Posner KL, Lee LA, Caplan RA, Domino KB. Trends in anesthesia-related death and brain damage: A closed claims analysis. Anesthesiology. 2006;**105**(6):1081-1086

[3] Li G, Warner M, Lang BH, Huang L, Sun LS. Epidemiology of anesthesia-related mortality in the United States, 1999-2005. Anesthesiology. 2009;**110**(4):759-765

[4] Cook TM, Woodall N, Frerk C, Fourth National Audit Project. Major complications of airway management in the UK: Results of the fourth National Audit Project of the Royal College of Anaesthetists and the difficult airway society. Part 1: Anaesthesia. British Journal of Anaesthesia. 2011;**106**(5):617-631

[5] Echevarría-Correas MA, González-Bada A, Rodrigo-Casanova MP, García-Peña JM, Aguilera-Celorrio L. Vía aérea difícil, detección preoperatoria y manejo en quirófano. Revista Mexicana de Anestesiología. 2015;**38**(2):85-90

[6] Marisa Mariscal Flores, Eugenio Martínez Hurtado. Manual de manejo de la Vía Aérea Difícil [Internet]. Disponible en: https://shop.anestesiar.org/tienda/manual-vad-pdf/

[7] Elliott DSJ, Baker PA, Scott MR, Birch CW, Thompson JMD. Accuracy of surface landmark identification for cannula cricothyroidotomy. Anaesthesia. 2010;**65**(9):889-894

[8] Law JA, Duggan LV, Asselin M, Baker P, Crosby E, Downey A, et al. Canadian airway focus group updated consensus-based recommendations for management of the difficult airway: Part 2. Planning and implementing safe management of the patient with an anticipated difficult airway. Canadian Journal of Anaesthesia. 2021;**68**(9):1405-1436

[9] Law JA, Duggan LV, Asselin M, Baker P, Crosby E, Downey A, et al. Canadian airway focus group updated consensus-based recommendations for management of the difficult airway: Part 1. Difficult airway management encountered in an unconscious patient. The Canadian Journal of Anesthesia. 2021;**68**(9):1373-1404

[10] Hung O, Murphy M. Context-sensitive airway management. Anesthesia and Analgesia. 2010;**110**(4):982-983

[11] Ahmad I, El-Boghdadly K, Bhagrath R, Hodzovic I, McNarry AF, Mir F, et al. Difficult airway society guidelines for awake tracheal intubation (ATI) in adults. Anaesthesia. 2019;**75**(5):688

[12] Cabrini L, Baiardo Redaelli M, Ball L, Filippini M, Fominskiy E, Pintaudi M, et al. Awake Fiberoptic intubation protocols in the operating room for anticipated difficult airway: A systematic review and meta-analysis of randomized controlled trials. Anesthesia & Analgesia. 2019;**128**(5):971-980

[13] Frerk C, Mitchell VS, McNarry AF, Mendonca C, Bhagrath R, Patel A, et al. Difficult airway society 2015 guidelines for management of unanticipated difficult intubation in adults. British Journal of Anaesthesia. 2015;**115**(6):827-848

[14] Apfelbaum JL, Hagberg CA, Connis RT, Abdelmalak BB, Agarkar M, Dutton RP, et al. American Society of Anesthesiologists Practice Guidelines for management of the difficult airway. Anesthesiology. 2022, 2022;**136**(1):31-81

[15] Murphy M, Hung O, Launcelott G, Law JA, Morris I. Predicting the difficult laryngoscopic intubation: Are we on the right track? Canadian Journal of Anesthesia. 2005;**52**(3):231-235

[16] Galán Gutiérrez JC, Mora PC, Pestana AS. Inducción inhalatoria y anestesia tópica de la vía aérea guiada por videolaringoscopio C-MAC pala d-Blade en un paciente con miastenia gravis y vía aérea difícil. Revista Colombiana de Anestesiología [Internet]. 2023;**41**:287-290. Disponible en: https://www.elsevier.es/es-revista-revista-colombiana-anestesiologia-341-articulo-induccion-inhalatoria-anestesia-topica-via-S0120334713000397?referer=coleccion

[17] Fernandez-Vaquero MA, Charco-Mora P, Garcia-Aroca MA, Greif R. Preoperative airway ultrasound assessment in the sniffing position: a prospective observational study. Brazilian Journal of Anesthesiology (English Edition). Jul 2022

[18] Wieczorek PM, Backman SB. Airway topical anesthesia. Anesthesia and Analgesia. 2009;**109**(3):991; author reply 991-992

[19] Pintaric TS. Upper airway blocks for awake difficult airway management. Acta Clinica Croatica. 2016;**55**(Suppl. 1):85-89

[20] Novitch M, Prabhakar A, Siddaiah H, Sudbury AJ, Kaye RJ, Wilson KE, et al. Point of care ultrasound for the clinical anesthesiologist. Best Practice & Research. Clinical Anaesthesiology. 2019;**33**(4):433-446

[21] Umobong EU, Mayo PH. Critical care airway management. Critical Care Clinics. 2018;**34**(3):313-324

[22] Fernández-Vaquero MÁ, Carrillo-Esper R. Ecografía de vía aérea: en busca de la membrana cricotiroidea. Revista Mexicana de Anestesiología. 2021;**44**(2):116-122

[23] Krause M, Khatibi B, Sztain JF, Rahman P, Shapiro AB, Sandhu NS. Ultrasound-guided airway blocks using a curvilinear probe. Journal of Clinical Anesthesia. 2016;**33**:408-412

[24] Iida T, Suzuki A, Kunisawa T, Iwasaki H. Ultrasound-guided superior laryngeal nerve block and translaryngeal block for awake tracheal intubation in a patient with laryngeal abscess. Journal of Anesthesia. 2013;**27**(2):309-310

[25] Manikandan S, Neema PK, Rathod RC. Ultrasound-guided bilateral superior laryngeal nerve block to aid awake endotracheal intubation in a patient with cervical spine disease for emergency surgery. Anaesthesia and Intensive Care. 2010;**38**(5):946-948

[26] Minogue SC, Ralph J, Lampa MJ. Laryngotracheal topicalization with lidocaine before intubation decreases the incidence of coughing on emergence from general anesthesia. Anesthesia and Analgesia. 2004;**99**(4):1253-1257

[27] Tanaka Y, Nakayama T, Nishimori M, Sato Y, Furuya H. Lidocaine for preventing postoperative sore throat. Cochrane Database of Systematic Reviews. 2009;**3**:CD004081

[28] Tsui B, Ip V, Walji A. Airway sonography in live models and cadavers. Journal of Ultrasound in Medicine. 2013;**32**(6):1049-1058

[29] Kaur B, Tang R, Sawka A, Krebs C, Vaghadia H. A method for

ultrasonographic visualization and injection of the superior laryngeal nerve: Volunteer study and cadaver simulation. Anesthesia and Analgesia. 2012;**115**(5):1242-1245

[30] Sawka A, Tang R, Vaghadia H. Sonographically guided superior laryngeal nerve block during awake fiberoptic intubation. A A Case Reports. 2015;**4**(8):107-110

[31] Rodríguez-Martín C, de la Cruz RC, Ruiz Piñero M, Guerrero Peral ÁL. Refractory neuralgia of the superior laryngeal nerve: A case study. Neurología. 2016;**31**(5):344-345

[32] Kristensen MS. Ultrasonography in the management of the airway. Acta Anaesthesiologica Scandinavica. 2011;**55**(10):1155-1173

[33] Barberet G, Henry Y, Tatu L, Berthier F, Besch G, Pili-Floury S, et al. Ultrasound description of a superior laryngeal nerve space as an anatomical basis for echoguided regional anaesthesia. British Journal of Anaesthesia. 2012;**109**(1):126-128

[34] Kumar A, Sinha C, Kumar A, Bhadani UK. Transverse approach for ultrasound-guided superior laryngeal nerve block for awake fiberoptic intubation. Saudi Journal of Anaesthesia. 2017;**11**(3):373-374

[35] Simmons ST, Schleich AR. Airway regional anesthesia for awake fiberoptic intubation. Regional Anesthesia and Pain Medicine. 2002;**27**(2):180-192

Chapter 3

Novel Techniques and Local Anesthetics for Perioperative Pain Management

Ashley Wang, Katrina Kerolus, Evan Garry, Deborah Li, Amruta Desai and Sergio Bergese

Abstract

Careful perioperative pain management is crucial for good patient outcomes after surgery, as poorly controlled pain interferes with the ability of patients to recover to normal baseline function and increases postoperative morbidity and mortality. Although opioids have been the mainstay for treating postoperative pain, there has been a shift in favor of a multimodal analgesic approach, including regional anesthesia, as a way to circumvent opioid-related adverse events (e.g. nausea and vomiting, respiratory depression, sedation). In this chapter, we present an update on several recently developed regional anesthetic techniques, local anesthetic medications, as well as nerve block adjuncts with the potential to improve pain management in the perioperative setting. With more future studies, these novel methods may be incorporated into postsurgical recovery protocols and provide the opportunity to improve patient outcomes.

Keywords: regional anesthesia, nerve blocks, erector spinae plane block (ESPB), pericapsular nerve group (PENG) block, interspace between the popliteal artery and posterior capsule of the knee (iPACK) block, genicular block, external oblique intercostal block, long-acting local Anesthetics, block adjuncts

1. Introduction

Prevention, treatment, and management of pain are crucial to delivering good outcomes for patients undergoing surgery. Poorly controlled pain from surgeries can trigger physiological stress responses that damage body organs while causing psychological and emotional distress to patients, thereby increasing postoperative morbidity and mortality [1]. Additionally, inadequate pain control may also interfere with the ability of patients to participate in rehabilitation activities, prolong length of hospitalization, and raise the overall cost of healthcare [2, 3]. Historically, opioids have been the mainstay for postoperative pain. However, to avoid the myriad of opioid-related adverse events (e.g. respiratory depression, sedation, vomiting), there has been a shift in favor of multimodal analgesia in recent years to combine different classes of analgesics and create a synergistic effect to alleviate pain [1, 4]. One major component of multimodal analgesia is regional anesthesia and nerve blocks to reduce perioperative pain. In this chapter, we present several novel regional anesthesia techniques, local anesthetic medications, and nerve block adjuncts developed in recent years that offer unique advantages for pain management in the perioperative setting. Further future research to investigate these techniques and medications will be critical for developing evidence-based guidelines and protocols in order to improve patient outcomes in surgical settings.

2. Erector spinae plane block (ESPB)

The erector spinae plane block (ESPB) is a relatively novel regional technique for acute and chronic pain management which delivers local anesthetics between the thoracic transverse process and the erector spinae muscles [5, 6]. The ESPB was first described by Forero et al. in 2016 as an ultrasound-guided interfascial plane block that not only produces effective multi-dermatomal analgesia for severe chronic neuropathic pain from metastatic disease of the ribs and rib fractures, but also improves postoperative pain in patients undergoing video-assisted thoracoscopic lobectomies [5]. Since then, the ESPB has gained popularity for its simplicity, safety, and ease of delivery. Its use for perioperative pain management has expanded to a wide variety of surgeries, including thoracotomies [7], breast surgeries [7, 8], ventral hernia repair [9], percutaneous nephrolithotomies [10], and even lumbar fusion [11–13].

2.1 Anatomy and technique

The ESPB mainly involves the deep intrinsic back muscles, which are divided into three layers: spinotransversales (superficial), erector spinae muscles (intermediate), and transversospinales (deep) [6, 14]. The spinotransversales layer allows for neck extension and head rotation, whereas the intermediate erector spinae muscles are a complex muscular group that connects the spinous processes, ribs, and transverse processes from each side of the spine. Finally, the transversospinales layer deep to the erector spinae muscles joins the transverse processes to the spinous processes [6, 14].

As each upper thoracic spinal nerve exits the intervertebral foramen, it separates into the dorsal and ventral rami. The dorsal ramus runs posteriorly into the erector spinae muscle before splitting to lateral and medial branches. The medial branch continues posteriorly to supply a posterior cutaneous branch for the back of the chest. On the other hand, the ventral ramus curves laterally to become the intercostal nerve. It gives rise to the lateral cutaneous branch at the angle of the rib to innervate the lateral chest, as well as the anterior cutaneous branch supplying the anterior chest wall and upper abdomen [5, 14]. The way the ESPB achieves relief of the bony neuropathic pain at the anterior, lateral, and posterior chest wall suggests that the local anesthetics must target both the dorsal and ventral rami of the thoracic spinal nerve [5, 6]. In other words, the best site of local anesthetic injection should be near the intervertebral foramina where the dorsal and ventral rami split deep (rather than superficial) to the erector spinae muscles [5, 6].

The precise mechanism of action for ESPBs, particularly regarding the pattern and variability of local anesthetic spread to the paravertebral spread, is still under investigation through studies on cadaveric models and in treated patients [6]. In thoracic ESPBs, Yang et al.'s cadaveric study reported consistent distribution of local anesthetics to the paravertebral space [15], whereas Ivanusic et al. found more dorsal ramus involvement but minimal spread of injected agent to the paravertebral space [16]. Other studies found that the extent of local anesthetic spread to the paravertebral space may depend on the level of the block [17] or the volume of injection [18]. Further studies are warranted to better understand the distribution of local anesthetics and improve the efficacy of ESPBs.

The key steps to a successful ESPB are identifying the transverse process and positioning of the needle tip for proper local anesthetic delivery [6]. It is most commonly done at the T5-T7 levels, though lumbar ESPBs have become more widely used in recent years. First, the patient is put in a seated position before a linear ultrasound transducer is placed longitudinally and about 3 cm lateral to the target spinal level. This allows one to obtain a parasagittal view of the trapezius, rhomboid major, and erector spinae muscles superficial to the hyperechoic spinous process [5, 6]. The block needle is then inserted in either a cephalad-to-caudad or caudad-to-cephalad direction until the tip reaches the interfascial layer between the rhombus major and erector spinae muscles, preferably deep to the erector spinae muscles. Upon injection of a bolus of local anesthetic, one should observe a linear separation of fluid between the muscle layers, confirming proper positioning [5, 6, 14]. Typically, 20–30 mL of 0.25% bupivacaine or 0.5% ropivacaine are used. An indwelling catheter may be inserted for continuous infusion or intermittent boluses [5, 14].

2.2 Clinical indications and trials

The ESPB is most commonly used for thoracic procedures. In a systemic review of randomized trials comparing thoracic ESPBs to sham or no block, Saadawi et al. noted that treatment with ESPBs led to reduced postoperative opioid consumptions as well as lower pain scores [6]. These results were reflected in a variety of surgeries, from breast cancer surgery [19] and mastectomy [20] to laparoscopic cholecystectomy [21], splenectomy [22], and open epigastric hernia repair [23]. In a meta-analysis looking specifically at thoracic and breast surgeries, Huang et al. also concluded improvement of postoperative analgesia from ESPBs as well as lower rate of postoperative nausea and vomiting (PONV) compared to no blocks [7]. Furthermore, Huang et al. found that the analgesic efficacy of ESPBs to be comparable to that of thoracic paravertebral blocks (TPVB). The analysis showed no significant overall difference in postoperative pain scores or in incidence of PONV between ESPBs and TPVB [7]. Since it targets a plane further from the pleura and neuraxial structures compared to TPVB, the ESPB may be a promising alternative block with lower risks of pleural puncture and local anesthetic systemic toxicity.

Spinal surgeries have been associated with high postoperative pain scores [24]. Whereas conventional opioid-based analgesia is associated with many opioid-related adverse events (e.g. nausea, vomiting, sedation), the rise of multimodal analgesic—which includes regional anesthesia—allows for improved management of postoperative pain in spinal surgeries. ESPBs. Systemic reviews and meta-analyses have examined randomized controlled trials (RCTs) comparing ESPBs with no block following lumbar spine surgeries, including lumbar decompression surgery, lumbar discectomy, and lumbar internal fixation [12, 13]. These studies have found that patients who had ESPBs in the perioperative period reported lower postoperative pain scores both at rest and with movement for 48 hours after surgery. In addition, ESPB patients consumed less opioids postoperatively, had lower incidence of PONV, and required shorter length of hospital stay. Additional analysis noted further reduction in postoperative opioid use for ESPBs performed at level of incision or operation rather than at fixed level [13]. While the current meta-analyses found that the ESPB provided effective postoperative analgesia in spine surgeries, future studies with higher quality evidence are warranted to confirm the clinical significance and possible superiority of ESP.

While most commonly used in thoracic surgeries, the ESPB also enhances pain management for renal procedures. Adequate analgesia in renal procedures requires the blockade of both somatic and visceral nerves innervating the skin, muscle, kidneys, and ureters. Given that renal pain transmits from the T10 to L1 level, the ESPB offers a promising solution. In a 2019 single-blinded RCT including 50 patients, Ibrahim et al. evaluated the analgesic efficacy of the ESPB compared to no block for percutaneous nephrolithotomy (PCNL) [10]. The block was performed in a single-shot at the T11 level unilaterally. The results showed lower intraoperative fentanyl consumption, lower morphine use 24 h after surgery, and higher rates of patient satisfaction for the treatment group. In addition, Ibrahim et al. noted statistically significant lower pain scale scores at 2 and 12 h in the ESPB group, though with only 1-point lower in pain scores compared to the control which may not be clinically relevant. A RCT study with 60 patients by Abdelgalil et al. compared the ESPB at the T7 level with patient-controlled analgesia (PCA) in open nephrectomy for renal malignancies, showing similar results of lower intraoperative and postoperative opioid consumption for the ESPB group [25]. Furthermore, Abdelgalil et al. found lower pain scores both at rest and with movement in the ESPB group, with a more clinically significant 2-point difference minimum in pain scores with movement in the first 24 h postoperatively compared to the control.

The use of ESPB has been expanded to address pain from the shoulder and upper extremity. A case series by Ma et al. reported successful analgesia with cervical ESPB (performed at the C6 or C7 level) for six patients undergoing shoulder arthroscopy, an intervention for severe rotator cuff injuries typically associated with severe postoperative pain [26]. The study reported that four out of the six patients did not require supplemental postoperative analgesia and that all were able to be discharged home safely the day after surgery. Similarly, a case report by Lee et al. demonstrated the use of ESPB in the emergency department setting for a patient with chronic radicular left arm pain limiting range of motion of the shoulder and elbow despite over-the-counter medications, topical patches, acupuncture, and a variety of other interventions [27]. Lee et al. noted complete relief of pain symptoms and restoration of range of motion for the patient 30 min after receiving the ESPB at the T2 level. The patient also reported complete pain relief for 5 days, with gradual return of symptoms at a more tolerable level afterwards. Together, these preliminary findings presented the ESPB as a potential regional anesthesia technique for upper limb injuries with lower risk of diaphragmatic paresis, upper extremity motor paresis, and nerve injury compared to the more widely used brachial plexus block.

3. Pericapsular nerve group (PENG) block

The pericapsular nerve group (PENG) block is a novel ultrasound-guided regional anesthesia technique that targets the articular branches to the anterior hip joint capsule—namely the femoral nerve (FN) and accessory obturator nerve (AON)—which is the most richly innervated part of the joint [28, 29]. When it was first described by Girón-Arango in 2018, the PENG block was used in perioperative pain management for hip fracture patients undergoing surgical reduction and fixation [28]. The PENG block serves as an alternative to other regional analgesic techniques such as the femoral nerve block (FNB) or fascial iliaca block (FIB) which are popular for hip procedures, with the added advantage of accessory obturator and the obturator nerves block coverage [28].

3.1 Anatomy and technique

Sensory innervation to the anterior hip joint capsule is provided by three nerves: the femoral nerve (FN), obturator nerve (ON), and accessory obturator nerve (AON). The FN, the largest branch of the lumbar plexus, originates from the ventral rami of L2 to L4 nerves and gives rise to the hip articular branches distal to the lateral border of the psoas muscle at around the L5 level which mostly innervate the lateral and superomedial portions of the hip capsule [29]. The ON begins at the ventral rami of the L2 to L4 nerves and passes through the obturator foramen before splitting into anterior and posterior branches at the thigh. The ON articular branches pass through the inferomedial (or "incisura") of the acetabulum between the pubic and ischial bones to supply the inferomedial area of the hip capsule [29]. Finally, the AON, present in 8–29% of the population [30], originates from the ventral rami of L3 to L4 nerves and descends along the medial border of the psoas major muscle past the superior ramus of the pubis and under the pectineus muscle before splitting into further branches. These AON branches supply the pectineus muscle and join the anterior branches of the ON at the medial aspect of the hip capsule [29].

Past studies have identified FN, ON, and AON as the major nerves of the hip joint, with ON and AON being reported as the most common source of innervation. However, a major cadaveric study in 2017 by Short et al. which included 13 specimens has found consistent innervation of the anterior hip capsule by FNs and ONs specifically, whereas AON branches were found to be less significant contributors [31]. Short et al. also identified pertinent anatomical landmarks for finding the articular branches of the hip joint: the "teardrop" bone thickening of the inferomedial acetabulum for ON, the anterior superior iliac spine (AIIS), and the iliopubic eminence (IPE) for FN and AON [31]. These findings inspired Giron et al. to develop the PENG block in order to more effectively target the FN and AON between the AIIS and IPE [28, 32].

To perform the PENG block, a patient is typically positioned supine with hip extended. For the in-plane technique, a curvilinear ultrasound probe is placed in a transverse plane over the AIIS before rotating 30–45 degrees to align with pubic ramus. This allows one to visualize the iliopsoas muscle and tendon sitting on the IPE along with the femoral artery and the more medial pectineus muscle. Next, a 22-gauge needle may be inserted in a lateral-to-medial in-plane approach to aim the tip in the plane between the psoas tendon anteriorly and the pubic ramus posteriorly. After needle positioning and negative aspiration, a volume of 8–30 mL of local anesthetics (e.g. bupivacaine, ropivacaine, or lidocaine) may be injected for analgesia [28, 32]. With the out-of-plane technique, the ultrasound probe is placed at the level of the anterior superior iliac spine (ASIS) parallel to the inguinal fold then rotated median until the upper pubic ramus is visible. As a result, the target area of local anesthetic injection, i.e. the area between the psoas muscle with a prominent tendon and the pubic ramus, may be located and approached out-of-plane.

3.2 Clinical indications and trials

The PENG block is most commonly used for hip-related analgesia, such as in the setting of hip fractures, pelvic fractures, and hip surgeries. While initial review studies have identified the PENG block as a promising alternative to other regional techniques (e.g. FNB, FIB), most of the evidence was limited to case reports and case series only [33]. In the last 2 years, there has been a rise in randomized controlled studies that strive to examine the safety and efficacy of PENG blocks in order to improve understanding of the novel technique.

When compared against sham placebo blocks or no blocks in total hip arthroplasty (THA), the results on the PENG block were mixed. Pascarella et al. found a significant reduction in opioid consumption, enhanced range of hip motion, and shortened time to ambulation after surgery with PENG block treatment [34], whereas Zheng et al. noted mostly short-term benefits (e.g. reduced intraoperative opioid dosing, lower maximal pain score in recovery room, fewer incidence of PONV) but no notable difference in outcomes upon discharge from recovery (e.g. no difference in pain score or muscle strength) [35]. On the other hand, Amato et al. found no improvement in analgesia for the PENG block treatment group compared to the sham block group after hip arthroscopy [36].

There have been several RTCs comparing the PENG block against FIB in the setting of hip arthroplasty. In terms of postoperative pain level, most RTCs reported little to no difference in pain scores at rest or with movement 48 h after the surgery between the PENG block and FIB groups [37–39]. Similarly, most studies found no notable difference in the cumulative postoperative opioid consumption or overall length of hospital stay [37–39]. However, this may vary based on patient condition and demographics. For example, the RCT by Hua et al. specifically examined the analgesic effect of the PENG block in elderly patients (ages 65–85) with femoral neck fracture; they found significantly lower dynamic and static pain scores in the PENG block group, as well as higher patient satisfaction score compared to the FIB group [40].

Several RCTs also looked at the level of postoperative motor function between the two groups [37–38, 40]. While Choi did not observe differences in quadriceps strength of either the operative or nonoperative legs in the PENG block group versus the FIB group, Aliste et al. found lower incidence of quadriceps motor block (i.e. paresis or paralysis of knee extension) at 3 and 6 h after the procedure in the PENG block group, as well as better hip adduction and thigh sensory function [38]. Similarly, Hua et al.'s study on the elderly population reported quadricep weakness in the FIB group but none from the PENG block group [40]. These results were also reflected in Liang et al.'s study in which the PENG block was combined with lateral femoral cutaneous nerve (LFCN) block. Liang et al. found that the combination of PENG with LFCN blocks led to earlier first postoperative walking time, greater degree of hip flexion, and stronger muscle strength compared to FIB, making the combined block a good candidate for enhanced recovery programs [39]. Overall, the preservation of motor function in PENG blocks offers the advantage of early postoperative ambulation and potentially quicker physical rehabilitation to normal activities.

4. Interspace between the popliteal artery and posterior capsule of the knee (iPACK) block

The interspace between the popliteal artery and posterior capsule of the knee (iPACK) block is an emerging analgesic method for total knee arthroplasties (TKA). First introduced in 2012 by Dr. Sanjay Sinha at St Francis Hospital and Medical Center in Hartford, CT, the iPACK block offers an ultrasound-guided alternative approach to managing posterior knee pain after TKA [41]. Whereas traditional regional anesthetics such as sciatic nerve blocks are associated with delayed functional recovery and motor weakness, the iPACK block aims to provide pain relief while preserving motor function [42].

4.1 Anatomy and technique

The iPACK block specifically targets the distal branches of the sciatic nerve to diminish the occurrence of foot drop, a common complication associated with TKA [43]. At the same time, it addresses pain in the posterior knee region by spreading through the popliteal fossa to the genicular branch of the obturator nerve and the inferior branches of the tibial nerve-nerves that are key analgesic targets for knee surgery [42, 44]. A cadaveric study has demonstrated that injectate consistently surrounds the middle genicular artery and likely involves the articular sensory nerves surrounding the vessel, thereby suggesting a potential mechanism for the iPACK block [44].

The optimal location of iPACK needle site entry remains a subject of ongoing investigation. A RCT showed that a distal iPACK block may result in improved motor function compared to a proximal block above the femoral condyle [45]. The proximal block targets the superior medial and lateral genicular nerves above the femoral condyle, which do not disperse to the sciatic nerve of the popliteal plexus. On the other hand, an iPACK injection below the femoral condyle may spread more effectively to the intercondylar region, thus reaching the popliteal plexus innervating the intra-articular and posterior knee regions [45]. A potential explanation for this difference may be that proximal injections spread more anteromedially, whereas distal injections promote greater anterolateral spread [46]. Further studies are required to confirm the exact mechanism of action.

4.2 Clinical indications and trials

While the iPACK block offers promising results and has been implemented in postoperative care, clinical data remain relatively limited. However, several studies have investigated the safety and efficacy of the technique.

The use of the iPACK block is most commonly combined with adductor canal blocks (ACB) following TKA. Kertkaiatkachorn et al. observed patients receiving either continuous ACB with iPACK treatment versus continuous ACB with periarticular injection (PAI) as an analgesic regimen [47]. The RCT found no significant difference in postoperative pain scores between the two groups. However, the iPACK block group demonstrated an increased IV morphine requirement compared to those in the PAI group. In addition, the iPACK group demonstrated a lower level of immediate ambulatory ability compared to the PAI group, though functional performance recovered with time [47].

Another study by Mou et al. compared three groups of patients receiving ACB and iPACK block, ACB only, and iPACK block only [48]. While patients receiving both ACB and iPACK block reported the lowest pain scores within 8 h postoperatively, those receiving iPACK block only reported the highest pain scores after 12–24 h as well as highest opioid consumption during hospitalization. No significant difference in postoperative complications or function evaluation was observed among the groups. These results suggest that while iPACK may reduce early pain when combined with ACB, the combination may not be clinically significant [48].

A systemic review by D'Souza et al. including eight RCTs (777 patients) assessed whether receiving an iPACK block as an adjunct after TKA would improve patient outcomes [49]. The analysis revealed that the majority of patients who received the adjunct iPACK block experienced no difference in postoperative opioid consumption, level of satisfaction, hospital length of stay, gait distance, and knee range of motion compared to those without iPACK block treatment. Similarly, a meta-analysis of

14 clinical trials (1044 patients) found that an iPACK block with ACB regimen did not improve postoperative pain at 6 hours in the presence of periarticular local infiltration analgesia (LIA) [50]. However, administering an iPACK block as an adjunct to ACB did provide better pain relief when periarticular LIA was not given. Overall, these results suggest that the iPACK block might not add significant clinical benefit as an adjunct.

While the iPACK block was originally intended for use after TKA, clinicians have begun exploring its use after anterior cruciate ligament (ACL) reconstruction. Martin et al. compared the combination of femoral triangle block and iPACK block to local infiltration analgesia after ACL reconstruction [51]. The results showed that even though the iPACK block treatment reduced consumption of morphine 24 h after surgery, it provided no notable difference in outcomes for analgesia or function [51]. This study is one of the few trials that studied iPACK blocks for a non-TKA surgery, suggesting the possibility for the block to be used in ACL reconstruction procedures. A case series has reflected similar results for using iPACK blocks after ACL reconstruction specifically in adolescent patients [52]. The three patients in the study reported minimal pain and no unexpected weakness in dorsiflexion or plantarflexion after receiving only one iPACK block postoperatively. The patients also required very little or no morphine after the procedure; the report confirmed that the iPACK blocks may be safely administered to adolescent patients undergoing ACL reconstruction.

Overall, current literature suggests that while iPACK may offer safe and effective anesthesia for postoperative posterior knee pain, it may not provide meaningful clinical benefits beyond those of standard of care. Although initially meant for use after TKA, the iPACK block may also be useful for ACL reconstruction. Further studies are necessary to better characterize the benefits of iPACK blocks, such as whether to be administered alone or with other analgesic techniques and its efficacy for other types of surgeries.

5. Genicular nerve block and cryoneurolysis for knee

Genicular nerve blocks involve many different branches of nerves from the femoral, saphenous, common fibular, and tibial nerves to innervate the joint capsule. This procedure was first developed to help with chronic knee pain and was later adopted for surgical procedures such as total knee arthroplasty [53]. Genicular nerve block selectively blocks articular branches and is motor-sparing. This can be potentially helpful in early ambulation and faster discharge of the patient following total knee replacement. Genicular nerve block and ablation have also been used as a successful modality in the management of chronic pain from knee osteoarthritis [54].

On the other hand, the use of cryoneurolysis, an opioid-sparing therapy in which cryoprobes freeze peripheral nerves, is becoming increasingly popular [55]. Cryoneurolysis causes nerves to undergo Wallerian degeneration, allowing relief from pain for up to 90 days as nerves regenerate [56, 57]. The device for the procedure utilizes liquid nitrous oxide being converted to a gas, generating a temperature of −125°C [58]. The advantages of cryoneurolysis include increased functional capacity and improved quality of life secondary to pain relief and ability to participate in physical exercise [59].

5.1 Anatomy

The knee is innervated by several different branches around the joint. The various nerves include nerve to vastus medialis (NVM), nerve to vastus lateralis (NVL), nerve to vastus intermedius (NVI), saphenous nerve (SN), common fibular nerve (CFN), recurrent fibular nerve (RFN), superolateral genicular nerve (SLGN), superomedial genicular nerve (SMGN), inferolateral genicular nerve (ILGN), and inferomedial genicular nerve (IMGN) [60]. There is variation in the exact trajectory of the genicular nerves, but the general landmarks around the nerves are fairly consistent across the population. Innervation of the joint capsule can be divided into four main quadrants: superolateral, superomedial, inferolateral, inferomedial.

5.2 Genicular nerve blocks

To perform the genicular nerve block, the patient is placed supine with his or her leg out straight and a pillow placed under the popliteal fossa [53]. Under ultrasound guidance, the articular branches of SMGN, SLGN, and IMGN are identified along the periosteum. There is the option to confirm the correct site for each using a peripheral nerve stimulation needle tip with nerve stimulation [61].

The SMGN starts in the superior popliteal region, tracks around the femur shaft, follows the superior medial genicular artery, then goes between the adductor magnus tendon and the medial epicondyle which is the target location for the block [62]. The superomedial genicular artery should be visible and courses along medially to the SMGN [61]. The SLGN runs laterally along the femur with the superolateral genicular artery and passes between the lateral epicondyle and vastus lateralis. The superolateral genicular artery is found between the vastus lateralis deep fascia and the femur, which is next to the target of the block and lateral to the SLGN [61, 62]. The IMGN lies between the medial tibial condyle and the shaft of the tibia. The inferomedial genicular artery can be seen inferior to the medial collateral ligament and inferomedial to the IMGN target [61]. The ILGN begins in the inferior popliteal region and courses around the tibial lateral epicondyle deep to the lateral collateral ligament, following the inferior lateral genicular artery superior to the fibula head [62]. It lies lateral and distal to the knee in a similar distribution to the RFN. Once each target nerve is identified, a 22-gauge needle can be introduced until bony contact is made with the femur, and 4–5 mL of long-acting local anesthetic (bupivacaine or ropivacaine) may be injected to the area.

The major limiting factor for the genicular nerve block is the fact that the genicular nerve is small while its trajectory is variable. As such, the block is mainly done based on bony landmarks with ultrasound guidance [63]. The option block for the ILGN, which is near the CFN, can lead to inadvertent postoperative foot drop, which may result in an extended time in the hospital waiting for the block to wear off. Due to the proximity to blood vessels and joints, there is an implicit risk of vascular or intra-articular puncture [62, 63].

5.3 Cryoneurolysis

Cryoneurolysis is the application of low temperatures (−20°C to −100°C) to a target percutaneous peripheral nerve to induce Wallerian degeneration; this subsequently disrupts the nerve function while nerve structure remains intact [56, 64]. Since nerve structure remains intact, this allows for complete nerve regeneration and a functional salvage of the nerve over time [65, 66]. Cryoneurolysis provides nonopioid pain relief with a lower risk of infection and no potential for local anesthetic toxicity or catheter dislodgement/leakage commonly seen with other pain management techniques. Additionally, there is a wide margin of safety with cryoanalgesia exceeding traditional local anesthetic-based peripheral nerve blocks, thereby enhancing its clinical utility [67]. The modern cryoprobes utilize gas (usually carbon dioxide or nitrous oxide) to generate extremely low temperatures. The cryoprobes consist of a hollow tube ranging from 1.4 mm to 2 mm with a smaller inner tube that injects pressurized gas at 600–800 psi [68].

Cryoneurolysis can be performed days prior to the proposed surgery. The patient is positioned supine with the leg straightened out and a pillow under the popliteal fossa. The two target nerves are the anterior femoral cutaneous nerve (AFCN) and the infrapatellar branch of the saphenous nerve (IPBSN) [58, 69].

The AFCN courses in the fascia on top of the quadriceps tendon and deep to subcutaneous fat on the anterior aspect of the leg. The target location for AFCN is around 70 mm above the superior pole of the patella [58]. A line in the transverse plane is drawn across the length from the medial and lateral edges of the patella where the needles for the treatment can be placed [58].

The IPBSN runs along the joint capsule and anterior inferior to the head of the tibia. The target location for IPBSN is roughly 50 mm below the inferior pole of the patella just medial to the patellar tendon [58]. A line in the sagittal plane may be drawn across the tibia from the inferior edge of the patella to the tibial tubercle for placement of needles for the treatment [58].

Once the target nerves are located and local anesthetics are applied to the cutaneous tissues, the needles can transmit cooling and warming for around 50 s, starting from one edge of the line to another for six cycles. A series of 2–3 min of freezing with 30 s of defrosting between each cycle is recommended [70]. Patients often note a burning or tingling during treatment which confirms the correct location. The entire procedure takes approximately 15 min [58]. Many newer nerve cryoprobes have built-in nerve stimulators for localization of the nerve and thermistors to detect the temperature, allowing for a wide margin of safety for the devices [70].

There are few relative or absolute contraindications to cryoneurolysis, including anticoagulation, bleeding disorders, localized infection, cryoglobulinemia, cold urticaria, paroxysmal cold haemoglobinuria, and Raynaud's syndrome [67]. Cryoneurolysis is contraindicated when extremity muscle demonstrates extreme weakness, such as ablating the femoral nerve for analgesia following a knee surgery in which the weakened quadriceps muscle prevents postoperative ambulation [67]. Other risks include bleeding, bruising, and minimal damage to surrounding tissue as the tissue may adhere to the frozen probe [58, 68]. After the procedure, there may also be depigmentation or hyperpigmentation [68].

5.4 Comparison to other knee blocks and future research

There is a limited number of studies that directly compare the genicular nerve block or cryoneurolysis. However, one study demonstrated that interspace between the popliteal artery and capsule of the knee (iPACK) block and the genicular nerve block both significantly reduced postoperative pain with no difference in time to mobilization after surgery. In fact, the genicular block was found to provide better pain relief 4 and 8 hours postoperatively when the patient is ambulating [71]. A recent review article found no RCTs for genicular nerve blocks to date, despite preliminary studies demonstrating for postoperative pain [72].

New techniques and devices for cryoneurolysis are being tested that utilize local injection of a "cold slurry" containing normal saline with 15% glycerol from −5°C down to −9°C. This can minimize the limitations of the current cryoneurolysis devices [55]. There is also ongoing research to optimize probe design [73]. Development of newer types of local anesthetics may also impact the future of genicular blocks.

Total knee replacement is a major surgery associated with significant postoperative pain. Therefore, nerve blocks are often used prior to the surgery to alleviate pain and potentially reduce opioid use. Additionally, cryoneurolysis may also provide longer pain relief than standard knee blocks. The techniques for these two procedures are fairly easy and mostly landmarked-based rather than requiring direct visualization. Further research into the safety and efficacy of the two procedures will allow for better assessment and understanding of appropriate clinical application for patients.

6. External oblique intercostal block

The external oblique intercostal (EOI) block is a novel superficial plane regional anesthesia technique that offers promising benefits for postoperative analgesia in upper abdominal surgeries [74]. The external oblique muscle is the most superficial muscular layer of the abdominal wall. Covering the anterior and lateral parts of the abdomen, it attaches to the lower eight ribs and runs inferiorly, medially, and anteriorly, ending midline at the linea alba [75]. It is innervated by the motor branches of the lateral cutaneous branches of anterior spinal nerves from T5 to T12 [76]. A limited cadaveric study revealed that dye injections to the site of EOI blocks effectively spread to both the anterior and lateral cutaneous branches of the T6/T7 to T10/T11 intercostal nerves; this distribution may explain the mechanism of EOI injection [75].

In patients, EOI blocks are performed with subjects lying supine; the sixth and tenth ribs are identified by ultrasound. The injection entry point is at the level of the sixth rib medial to the anterior axillary line. The needle is advanced in a superomedial-to-inferolateral direction, through the external oblique muscle, until the tip lies between the external oblique and intercostal muscles at the caudal end of the rib [75]. With the EOI block, patients should experience consistent sensory blockade of T6 to T9 at the midline and T6 to T10 at the anterior axillary line [75]. This technique has been shown to be effective in bariatric and liver surgery with patients having reduced opioid consumption and improved postoperative pain scores [77–79].

Obesity is associated with higher rates of complications and block failure. One challenge includes technical difficulties related to the depth of the target site [80, 81]. Obesity is an important consideration in regional anesthesia and often considered a contraindication for procedures such as paravertebral blockade, thoracic epidural analgesia, and erector spinae plane catheter insertion [81]. A case study reported successful administration of EOI block in two morbidly obese patients despite technical challenges [81]. This suggests the potential for EOI blocks to be used in a wider patient population compared to other regional analgesic methods. Future studies should further investigate the efficacy of EOI blocks in larger cohorts of obese patients in order to better understand the benefits, potential complications, and long-term outcomes of EOI blocks in this specific population.

In addition to its potential use for a wider patient population, the EOI block presents several advantages over other alternatives. For example, the transabdominal plane (TAP) blocks inconsistently block the innervation to the upper abdominal wall. Depending on the approach, subcostal TAP blocks typically cover either T6 to T7 or T10 to T11, but not both simultaneously [75]. In addition, unlike EOI blocks, TAP blocks often fail to block lateral cutaneous branches, thus limiting use in several abdominal surgical procedures [75, 82]. In contrast, EOI blocks seem to provide more for upper abdominal surgeries, though further research is needed to establish its efficacy, safety, and optimal application.

7. Long-acting local anesthetics and block adjuncts

Long-acting local anesthetics may be explored as potential solutions to improve analgesia and reduce postoperative opioids use. Traditional local anesthetics, such as lidocaine and bupivacaine, provide short- to intermediate-term pain relief. However, their duration of action is limited, leaving patients in pain once the effects subside and thus requiring other medications such as opioids for pain control.

Current research has focused on formulating new local anesthetics with liposomal or lipid-based delivery systems. The aim is to prolong the duration of analgesia, thereby reducing the need for additional pain interventions. These systems encapsulate the anesthetic drug, allowing for slow and sustained release over an extended period. By controlling the release rate, these formulations can provide analgesia for several days, significantly reducing the need for opioids postoperatively. Another strategy involves using novel compounds or modifying existing local anesthetics to enhance the duration of action. These modifications include adding additives in nerve blocks or altering the chemical structure of the drug to increase potency or delay metabolism, thereby extending the analgesic effects. Preliminary studies and clinical trials have shown promising results with some of these long-acting local anesthetics.

7.1 Liposomal bupivacaine

Liposomal bupivacaine, also known as extended-release bupivacaine, is similar to a micelle, creating a bilayer of lipids with bupivacaine inside the structure. In 2011, Bupivacaine liposome injectable suspension (Exparel) was approved as a local anesthetic by the US Food and Drug Administration (FDA) for single-dose infiltration in adults for postsurgical local anesthesia and for interscalene brachial plexus nerve blocks [83, 84]. The drug has a slower release than typical bupivacaine due to its liposomal structure which substantially prolongs the analgesic effects [85].

When liposomal bupivacaine is administered, the local anesthetic effect diminishes over time while the systemic levels of bupivacaine may persist for up to 96 h [86]. The prolonged effect makes liposomal bupivacaine beneficial for postoperative analgesia. To prevent unintentional overdose and systemic toxicity, one should avoid administering immediate-release bupivacaine or other local anesthetics for at least 96 h after liposomal bupivacaine use [86].

The evidence supporting the effectiveness of liposomal bupivacaine for postoperative pain management has been limited. A review by Ilfeld et al. looked at 12 placebo-controlled RCTs investigating liposomal bupivacaine infiltration into the surgical site for postoperative pain management after procedures in the trunk, extremities, and dentition [87]. Only five of the 12 RCTs demonstrated improved pain management from liposomal bupivacaine compared to the placebo control group [87]. Furthermore, Ilfeld et al. noted an increased risk of bias in all five RTCs [87–89]. When comparing liposomal bupivacaine to traditional bupivacaine hydrochloride, an older and shorter-acting analgesic, only two out of 19 RTCs reported statistically and clinically significant difference in postoperative pain scores for liposomal bupivacaine after various surgeries (excluding knee arthroplasty). Similarly, only two out of 17 RCTs for knee arthroplasty found a significant difference in pain scores and postoperative opioid use for the liposomal bupivacaine group compared to traditional bupivacaine [85, 87, 90, 91].

RTCs evaluating single-shot nerve blocks and continuous peripheral nerve blocks for knee and shoulder procedures found liposomal bupivacaine to be superior to typical anesthetics for pain control and reduced postoperative opioid consumption [87, 92–102]. However, RTCs on liposomal bupivacaine use in TAP blocks and epidural blocks after abdominal surgery showed mixed results; there was no difference in pain scores or postoperative opioid use between TAP block using liposomal bupivacaine compared to epidural blocks with fentanyl [103].

7.2 Bupivacaine/meloxicam

Bupivacaine/meloxicam (Zynrelef) is a combination drug in fixed doses of the local anesthetic, bupivacaine, and meloxicam. This is a prolonged-release formulation that lasts approximately 72 h and is applied with a needle-free technique into a surgical site where it can target local tissues just below the skin. Phase III clinical trials using bupivacaine/meloxicam in bunionectomies, herniorrhaphies, and total knee arthroplasty have demonstrated a statistically significant decrease in pain and opioid consumption compared to placebo and bupivacaine hydrochloride. Wound healing was not impacted, and adverse effects were similar to placebo [104].

7.3 Lidocaine infusion

The proposed benefits of continuous systemic lidocaine infusion in the perioperative setting is to reduce the need for opioids and inhaled anesthetic agents as well as allow for the return of bowel function after surgery to shorten the length of stay in the hospital [105]. A systematic review of 68 trials included studies that compared lidocaine infusion to thoracic epidural analgesia, placebo, or no treatment during general anesthesia cases that were either urgent or elective. The procedures studied included open abdominal and laparoscopic abdominal surgeries. Lidocaine infusion was started prior to the incision intraoperatively and continued until at least the end of the surgery. There was no clear evidence of improvement in pain scores, return of bowel function after surgery, or lower opioid consumption compared to placebo or no treatment. In addition, there was insufficient evidence for lidocaine infusion compared to epidural anesthesia since the studies varied in dosing and timing of the infusion [106].

7.4 Mepivacaine

Mepivacaine is an intermediate-acting local anesthetic with a shorter duration at around 1.5–2 h. Review articles of RCTs and retrospective cohort studies have compared mepivacaine and bupivacaine for spinal anesthesia in total hip arthroplasty and total knee arthroplasty [107, 108]. The results found that mepivacaine treatment is associated with higher incidence of complete motor blocks, shorter hospital stay, faster resolution of the motor block, sooner return to normal voiding function, and earlier time to ambulation compared to bupivacaine. However, mepivacaine also had higher incidences of transient neurologic symptoms and transient nerve root irritation than bupivacaine. There was no significant difference in pain scores or distance walked after surgery despite early ambulation with mepivacaine [107, 108].

In a meta-analysis that includes seven RTCs with 672 patients, Fu et al. compared mepivacaine and bupivacaine in combination blocks for the femoral and sciatic nerves, interscalene brachial plexus blocks, and spinal anesthesia [109]. Their findings showed that patients receiving mepivacaine experienced significantly faster return of motor function and shorter length of hospital stay. However, mepivacaine use was also associated with increased postoperative analgesic requirements such as opioids and nonsteroidal anti-inflammatory drugs (NSAIDs). This could be due to the shorter duration of action of mepivacaine, as well as early ambulation with mepivacaine leading to more pain from movement. Finally, no difference was found in postoperative pain scores, complications from blocks, or patient satisfaction between mepivacaine and bupivacaine [109].

7.5 Prilocaine

Prilocaine, a local anesthetic, has an intermediate length of duration with a fast onset of action. It is cleared faster than lidocaine and less likely to reach toxic blood levels, thus contributing to minimal side effects [110]. Prilocaine has been found to be particularly useful for spinal anesthesia in low doses [111]. Compared to bupivacaine, prilocaine use in obstetric anesthesia for cesarean sections was associated with a significantly reduced duration of the motor block and subsequently shorter stay in the post-anesthesia care unit [112]. Recently, 2% hyperbaric prilocaine has been approved for intrathecal use in Europe for 60- to 90-min procedures; however, it is only available for dental procedures in the US. While lidocaine may cause transient neurologic symptoms as a side effect in 10–40% of patients, intrathecal prilocaine may be a better option due to its lower incidence [111].

7.6 QX-OH/levobupivacaine (LL-1)

QX-OH is a quaternary lidocaine derivative shown to maintain local anesthetic effect over a long period in rats [113]. When QX-OH is combined with levobupivacaine (QX-OH/Levo-Bupi, or LL-1), the constant concentration ratio of 35 mM/10 mM was found to achieve the longest duration of action while having moderate local toxicity (QX-OH/Levo-Bupi, denoted as LL-1) [114]. This new combination in fixed-dose has shown good efficacy and fast onset of analgesia in animal models. Studies have shown that the two drugs create an additive effect of inhibition of sodium currents across cell membranes. In addition, LL-1 offers the advantage of low tissue toxicity in local injections [115–117]. Further investigation of LL-1 in human subjects is warranted.

7.7 Hydrogel/microsphere composite of bupivacaine and dexmedetomidine

A hydrogel/microsphere composite co-delivers local anesthetic bupivacaine in the microsphere and alpha-2 (a_2)-adrenergic receptor agonist dexmedetomidine in the hydrogel matrix; it was developed to prolong analgesia in single injections [118]. The goal was to release dexmedetomidine from the hydrogel and constrict surrounding local arteries to reduce bupivacaine uptake, similar to the role of epinephrine when combined with lidocaine for local anesthesia. Bupivacaine is released over a longer period to lengthen the duration of analgesia. Rat model studies of this extended-release drug formulation in sciatic nerve blocks have demonstrated a longer duration of nerve block while minimizing systemic toxicity from bupivacaine. This drug delivery system offers a viable strategy to extend the duration of single-shot nerve blocks for surgery [118].

7.8 Injectable electrospun fiber-hydrogel composite

An injectable regional anesthetic composite combining Rop-loaded electrospun nanofiber and Clo-loaded F127 hydrogel is a single-shot composite drug made of a poly-electrospun fiber of ε-caprolactone loaded with ropivacaine and F127 hydrogel loaded with clonidine [119]. Clonidine is released from the hydrogel to constrict neighboring local arteries while reducing ropivacaine uptake. Then, ropivacaine is slowly released over time to prolong blockage to the target area. Testing of the drug on rat models for sciatic nerve blocks showed the sensory and motor blocks lasting around 32 h and 20 h, respectively. This means a significant time with minimal pain and intact motor function. The injectable electrospun fiber-hydrogel composite may be useful for total knee arthroplasty and total hip arthroplasty [119].

7.9 Dexmedetomidine

Dexmedetomidine is a selective α_2-adrenoreceptor agonist which provides sedative, analgesic and anxiolytic properties. Clonidine, another adjunct which works on the same receptor, is eight times less specific for α_2-adrenoreceptor compared to dexmedetomidine [120]. The α_2-adrenoreceptor is a G-coupled protein widely found in the periphery, central nervous system and autonomic ganglion. When acting on the locus coeruleus nucleus, dexmedetomidine provides sedative and hypnotic effects. At the dorsal horn, it reduces the secretion of pain transmission molecules such as substance P and glutamate [121]. Dexmedetomidine also maintains the hyperpolarization state of interneurons by inhibiting I_h current. This leads to an amplified anesthetic effect on unmyelinated C pain fibers and small myelinated A-δ fibers which detect temperature and rapid pain sensation. In contrast, large myelinated motor fibers are less affected [122]. At lower doses, dexmedetomidine decreases heart rate and blood pressure by reducing vascular resistance. At larger and rapid doses, it is no longer selective, thereby causing increased blood pressure and decreased heart rate. Combining dexmedetomidine with local anesthetics in peripheral nerve blocks has demonstrated stronger analgesic effect and prolonged duration by 4–5 h compared to using local anesthetics alone [123]. This can be attributed to the drug's effect throughout the spinal cord, its ability to inhibit δ and C fibers and the vasoconstrictive properties leading to reduced absorption of local anesthetics [124]. In a meta-analysis looking at perineural dexmedetomidine in brachial plexus blocks, dexmedetomidine provided an increase in mean analgesia duration by 4.5 h–specifically 4 h of sensory block and 3 h of motor block. It also decreased the mean time onset for these blocks by 8–9 min. The optimal dose of perineural dexmedetomidine providing the longest sensory blockade with minimal adverse effects is 50–60 mcg [125]. Some adverse effects of dexmedetomidine to keep in mind are bradycardia, hypotension, and excessive sedation.

7.10 Intravascular and perineural dexamethasone

Dexamethasone is a long-acting glucocorticoid with minimal mineralocorticoid activity. It works as an anti-inflammatory by inhibiting cyclooxygenase-2 and prostaglandins. When administered perineurally, it is thought to increase inhibitory potassium channels, leading to decreased excitability and neuronal transmission in nociceptive unmyelinated C fibers responsible for pain [120]. Dexamethasone can be administered intravenously or perineurally to reduce postoperative pain and opioid consumption. Both routes as adjuncts have shown to prolong analgesia duration by approximately 6 h compared to the control group with no adjunct [125, 126]. In an meta-analysis testing the efficacy of perineural versus intravenous in brachial plexus blocks, the perineural route prolonged the duration of analgesia, sensory block, and motor block by approximately 132 min, 210 min, and 219 min respectively compared to intravenous dexamethasone [127]. Although perineural administration led to prolonged duration of action, many still recommend using IV dexamethasone at 0.1–0.2 mg/kg in patients undergoing moderate or severe surgeries because of its lower rates of PONV [128–130]. Discussion about the optimal dose for dexamethasone is still ongoing; some studies showed that perineural dexamethasone at high doses have no advantage but carry increased risk compared to lower doses. A randomized trial comparing 2, 5 and 8 mg perineural dexamethasone in infraclavicular blocks found similar durations of sensorimotor block [131]. Therefore, higher doses of perineural dexamethasone are no longer recommended. More studies to investigate the most effective dose for perineural dexamethasone are necessary.

Conflict of interest

The authors declare that the research was conducted in the absence of any commercial or financial relationships that could be construed as a potential conflict of interest.

Author details

Ashley Wang[1], Katrina Kerolus[1], Evan Garry[2], Deborah Li[2], Amruta Desai[1] and Sergio Bergese[1*]

1 Department of Anesthesiology, Stony Brook University Hospital, Stony Brook, NY, USA

2 Renaissance School of Medicine, Stony Brook University, Stony Brook, NY, USA

*Address all correspondence to: sergio.bergese@stonybrookmedicine.edu

References

[1] Joshi GP, Ogunnaike BO. Consequences of inadequate postoperative pain relief and chronic persistent postoperative pain. Anesthesiology Clinics of North America. 2005;**23**(1):21-36. DOI: 10.1016/j.atc.2004.11.013

[2] Apfelbaum JL, Chen C, Mehta SS, Gan TJ. Postoperative pain experience: Results from a national survey suggest postoperative pain continues to be undermanaged. Anesthesia and Analgesia. 2003;**97**(2):534-540. DOI: 10.1213/01.ANE.0000068822.10113.9E

[3] Gan TJ. Poorly controlled postoperative pain: Prevalence, consequences, and prevention. Journal of Pain Research. 2017;**10**:2287-2298. DOI: 10.2147/jpr.s144066

[4] Garimella V, Cellini C. Postoperative pain control. Clinics in Colon and Rectal Surgery. 2013;**26**(3):191-196. DOI: 10.1055/s-0033-1351138

[5] Forero M, Adhikary SD, Lopez H, Tsui C, Chin KJ. The erector spinae plane block: A novel analgesic technique in thoracic neuropathic pain. Regional Anesthesia and Pain Medicine. 2016;**41**(5):621-627. DOI: 10.1097/AAP.0000000000000451

[6] Saadawi M, Layera S, Aliste J, Bravo D, Leurcharusmee P, Tran DQ. Erector spinae plane block: A narrative review with systematic analysis of the evidence pertaining to clinical indications and alternative truncal blocks. Journal of Clinical Anesthesia. 2021;**68**(110063):110063. DOI: 10.1016/j.jclinane.2020.110063

[7] Huang W, Wang W, Xie W, Chen Z, Liu Y. Erector spinae plane block for postoperative analgesia in breast and thoracic surgery: A systematic review and meta-analysis. Journal of Clinical Anesthesia. 2020;**66**(109900):109900. DOI: 10.1016/j.jclinane.2020.109900

[8] Gürkan Y, Aksu C, Kuş A, Yörükoğlu UH. Erector spinae plane block and thoracic paravertebral block for breast surgery compared to IV-morphine: A randomized controlled trial. Journal of Clinical Anesthesia. 2020;**59**:84-88. DOI: 10.1016/j.jclinane.2019.06.036

[9] Chin KJ, Adhikary S, Sarwani N, Forero M. The analgesic efficacy of pre-operative bilateral erector spinae plane (ESP) blocks in patients having ventral hernia repair. Anaesthesia. 2017;**72**(4):452-460. DOI: 10.1111/anae.13814

[10] Ibrahim M, Elnabtity AM. Analgesic efficacy of erector spinae plane block in percutaneous nephrolithotomy: A randomized controlled trial: A randomized controlled trial. Der Anaesthesist. 2019;**68**(11):755-761. DOI: 10.1007/s00101-019-00673-w

[11] Singh S, Choudhary NK, Lalin D, Verma VK. Bilateral ultrasound-guided erector spinae plane block for postoperative analgesia in lumbar spine surgery: A randomized control trial: A randomized control trial. Journal of Neurosurgical Anesthesiology. 2020;**32**(4):330-334. DOI: 10.1097/ana.0000000000000603

[12] Ma J, Bi Y, Zhang Y, Zhu Y, Wu Y, Ye Y, et al. Erector spinae plane block for postoperative analgesia in spine surgery: A systematic review and meta-analysis. European Spine Journal. 2021;**30**(11):3137-3149. DOI: 10.1007/s00586-021-06853-w

[13] Oh SK, Lim BG, Won YJ, Lee DK, Kim SS. Analgesic efficacy of erector spinae plane block in lumbar spine surgery: A systematic review and meta-analysis. Journal of Clinical Anesthesia. 2022;**78**(110647):110647. DOI: 10.1016/j.jclinane.2022.110647

[14] De Cassai A, Bonvicini D, Correale C, Sandei L, Tulgar S, Tonetti T. Erector spinae plane block: A systematic qualitative review. Minerva Anestesiologica. 2019;**85**(3):308-319. DOI: 10.23736/S0375-9393.18.13341-4

[15] Yang H-M, Choi YJ, Kwon H-J, O J, Cho TH, Kim SH. Comparison of injectate spread and nerve involvement between retrolaminar and erector spinae plane blocks in the thoracic region: A cadaveric study. Anaesthesia. 2018;**73**(10):1244-1250. DOI: 10.1111/anae.14408

[16] Ivanusic J, Konishi Y, Barrington MJ. A cadaveric study investigating the mechanism of action of erector spinae blockade. Regional Anesthesia and Pain Medicine. 2018;**43**(6):567-571. DOI: 10.1097/aap.0000000000000789

[17] Dautzenberg KHW, Zegers MJ, Bleeker CP, Tan ECTH, Vissers KCP, van Geffen G-J, et al. Unpredictable injectate spread of the erector spinae plane block in human cadavers. Anesthesia and Analgesia. 2019;**129**(5):e163-e166. DOI: 10.1213/ANE.0000000000004187

[18] Choi Y-J, Kwon H-J, O J, Cho T-H, Won JY, Yang H-M, et al. Influence of injectate volume on paravertebral spread in erector spinae plane block: An endoscopic and anatomical evaluation. PLoS One. 2019;**14**(10):e0224487. DOI: 10.1371/journal.pone.0224487

[19] Aksu C, Kuş A, Yörükoğlu HU, Tor Kılıç C, Gürkan Y. Analgesic effect of the bi-level injection erector spinae plane block after breast surgery: A randomized controlled trial. Ağrı. 2019;**31**(3):132-137. DOI: 10.14744/agri.2019.61687

[20] Yao Y, Li H, He Q, Chen T, Wang Y, Zheng X. Efficacy of ultrasound-guided erector spinae plane block on postoperative quality of recovery and analgesia after modified radical mastectomy: Randomized controlled trial. Regional Anesthesia and Pain Medicine. 2019;**45**(1):5-9. DOI: 10.1136/rapm-2019-100983

[21] Aksu C, Kuş A, Yörükoğlu HU, Tor Kılıç C, Gürkan Y. The effect of erector spinae plane block on postoperative pain following laparoscopic cholecystectomy: A randomized controlled study. Anestezi Derg. 2019;**27**(1):9-14. DOI: 10.5222/jarss.2019.14632

[22] Mostafa SF, Abdelghany MS, Abdelraheem TM, Abu Elyazed MM. Ultrasound-guided erector spinae plane block for postoperative analgesia in pediatric patients undergoing splenectomy: A prospective randomized controlled trial. Paediatric Anaesthesia. 2019;**29**(12):1201-1207. DOI: 10.1111/pan.13758

[23] Abu Elyazed MM, Mostafa SF, Abdelghany MS, Eid GM. Ultrasound-guided erector spinae plane block in patients undergoing open epigastric hernia repair: A prospective randomized controlled study: A prospective randomized controlled study. Anesthesia and Analgesia. 2019;**129**(1):235-240. DOI: 10.1213/ANE.0000000000004071

[24] Gerbershagen HJ, Aduckathil S, van Wijck AJM, Peelen LM, Kalkman CJ, Meissner W. Pain intensity on the first day after surgery: A prospective cohort study comparing 179 surgical procedures. Anesthesiology. 2013;**118**(4):934-944. DOI: 10.1097/ALN.0b013e31828866b3

[25] Abdelgalil AS, Ahmed AM, Gamal RM, Elshal MM, Bakeer AH, Shaker EH. Ultrasound guided continuous erector spinae plane block versus patient controlled analgesia in open nephrectomy for renal malignancies: A randomized controlled study. Journal of Pain Research. 2022;**15**:3093-3102. DOI: 10.2147/JPR.S379721

[26] Ma D, Wang R, Wen H, Li H, Jiang J. Cervical erector spinae plane block as a perioperative analgesia method for shoulder arthroscopy: A case series. Journal of Anesthesia. 2021;**35**(3):446-450. DOI: 10.1007/s00540-021-02907-x

[27] Lee DH, Martel ML, Reardon RF. Erector spinae plane block in the emergency department for upper extremity: A case report. Clinical Practice and Cases in Emergency Medicine. 2021;**5**(3):353-356. DOI: 10.5811/cpcem.2021.3.51803

[28] Girón-Arango L, Peng PWH, Chin KJ, Brull R, Perlas A. Pericapsular nerve group (PENG) block for hip fracture. Regional Anesthesia and Pain Medicine. 2018;**43**(8):859-863. DOI: 10.1097/AAP.0000000000000847

[29] Del Buono R, Padua E, Pascarella G, Costa F, Tognù A, Terranova G, et al. Pericapsular nerve group block: An overview. Minerva Anestesiologica. 2021;**87**(4):458-466. DOI: 10.23736/S0375-9393.20.14798-9

[30] Archana B, Nagaraj D, Pradeep P, Subhash LP. Anatomical variations of accessory obturator nerve: A cadaveric study with proposed clinical implications. International Journal of Anatomy and Research. 2016;**4**(2):2158-2161. DOI: 10.16965/ijar.2016.168

[31] Short AJ, Barnett JJG, Gofeld M, Baig E, Lam K, Agur AMR, et al. Anatomic study of innervation of the anterior hip capsule: Implication for image-guided intervention. Regional Anesthesia and Pain Medicine. 2018;**43**:186-192. DOI: 10.1097/aap.0000000000000701

[32] Teles AS, Yamak Altınpulluk E, Sahoo RK, Galluccio F, Simón DG, İnce İ, et al. Beyond the pericapsular nerve group (PENG) block: A narrative review. The Turkish Journal of Anaesthesiology and Reanimation. 2022;**50**(3):167-172. DOI: 10.5152/TJAR.2021.21230

[33] Morrison C, Brown B, Lin D-Y, Jaarsma R, Kroon H. Analgesia and anesthesia using the pericapsular nerve group block in hip surgery and hip fracture: A scoping review. Regional Anesthesia and Pain Medicine. 2021;**46**(2):169-175. DOI: 10.1136/rapm-2020-101826

[34] Pascarella G, Costa F, Del Buono R, Pulitanò R, Strumia A, Piliego C, et al. Impact of the pericapsular nerve group (PENG) block on postoperative analgesia and functional recovery following total hip arthroplasty: A randomised, observer-masked, controlled trial. Anaesthesia. 2021;**76**(11):1492-1498. DOI: 10.1111/anae.15536

[35] Zheng J, Pan D, Zheng B, Ruan X. Preoperative pericapsular nerve group (PENG) block for total hip arthroplasty: A randomized, placebo-controlled trial. Regional Anesthesia and Pain Medicine. 2022;**47**(3):155-160. DOI: 10.1136/rapm-2021-103228

[36] Amato PE, Coleman JR, Dobrzanski TP, Elmer DA, Gwathmey FW Jr, Slee AE, et al. Pericapsular nerve group (PENG) block for hip arthroscopy: A randomized, double-blinded, placebo-controlled trial. Regional Anesthesia and Pain Medicine. 2022;**47**:728-732. DOI: 10.1136/rapm-2022-103907

[37] Choi YS, Park KK, Lee B, Nam WS, Kim D-H. Pericapsular nerve group (PENG) block versus supra-inguinal fascia iliaca compartment block for total hip arthroplasty: A randomized clinical trial. Journal of Personalized Medicine. 2022;**12**(3):408. DOI: 10.3390/jpm12030408

[38] Aliste J, Layera S, Bravo D, Jara Á, Muñoz G, Barrientos C, et al. Randomized comparison between pericapsular nerve group (PENG) block and suprainguinal fascia iliaca block for total hip arthroplasty. Regional Anesthesia and Pain Medicine. 2021;**46**(10):874-878. DOI: 10.1136/rapm-2021-102997

[39] Liang L, Zhang C, Dai W, He K. Comparison between pericapsular nerve group (PENG) block with lateral femoral cutaneous nerve block and supra-inguinal fascia iliaca compartment block (S-FICB) for total hip arthroplasty: A randomized controlled trial. Journal of Anesthesia. 2023;**37**:503-510. DOI: 10.1007/s00540-023-03192-6

[40] Hua H, Xu Y, Jiang M, Dai X. Evaluation of pericapsular nerve group (PENG) block for analgesic effect in elderly patients with femoral neck fracture undergoing hip arthroplasty. Journal of Healthcare Engineering. 2022;**2022**:7452716. DOI: 10.1155/2022/7452716

[41] Vlessides M. New regional technique controls post-TKA pain. In: Anesthesiology News. New York: McMahon Publishing; 2012. Available from: https://issuu.com/mcmahongroup/docs/mman0012_2012_tab

[42] Albrecht E, Wegrzyn J, Dabetic A, El-Boghdadly K. The analgesic efficacy of iPACK after knee surgery: A systematic review and meta-analysis with trial sequential analysis. Journal of Clinical Anesthesia. 2021;**72**(110305):110305. DOI: 10.1016/j.jclinane.2021.110305

[43] Thobhani S, Scalercio L, Elliott CE, Nossaman BD, Thomas LC, Yuratich D, et al. Novel regional techniques for total knee arthroplasty promote reduced hospital length of stay: An analysis of 106 patients. The Ochsner Journal. 2017;**17**(3):233-238

[44] Niesen AD, Harris DJ, Johnson CS, Stoike DE, Smith HM, Jacob AK, et al. Interspace between popliteal artery and posterior capsule of the knee (IPACK) injectate spread: A cadaver study: IPACK injectate spread. Journal of Ultrasound in Medicine. 2019;**38**(3):741-745. DOI: 10.1002/jum.14761

[45] Kampitak W, Tanavalee A, Ngarmukos S, Tantavisut S. Motor-sparing effect of iPACK (interspace between the popliteal artery and capsule of the posterior knee) block versus tibial nerve block after total knee arthroplasty: A randomized controlled trial. Regional Anesthesia and Pain Medicine. 2020;**45**(4):267-276. DOI: 10.1136/rapm-2019-100895

[46] Tran J, Giron Arango L, Peng P, Sinha SK, Agur A, Chan V. Evaluation of the iPACK block injectate spread: A cadaveric study. Regional Anesthesia and Pain Medicine. 2019;**44**(7):689-694. DOI: 10.1136/rapm-2018-100355

[47] Kertkiatkachorn W, Kampitak W, Tanavalee A, Ngarmukos S. Adductor canal block combined with iPACK (interspace between the popliteal artery and the capsule of the posterior knee) block vs periarticular injection for analgesia after total knee arthroplasty: A randomized noninferiority trial. The Journal of Arthroplasty. 2021;**36**(1):122-129.e1. DOI: 10.1016/j.arth.2020.06.086

[48] Mou P, Wang D, Tang X-M, Zeng W-N, Zeng Y, Yang J, et al. Adductor canal block combined with IPACK block for postoperative analgesia and function recovery following total knee arthroplasty: A prospective, double-blind, randomized controlled study. The Journal of Arthroplasty. 2022;**37**(2):259-266. DOI: 10.1016/j.arth.2021.10.004

[49] D'Souza RS, Langford BJ, Olsen DA, Johnson RL. Ultrasound-guided local anesthetic infiltration between the popliteal artery and the capsule of the posterior knee (IPACK) block for primary total knee arthroplasty: A systematic review of randomized controlled trials. Local. Regional Anesthesia. 2021;**14**:85-98. DOI: 10.2147/LRA.S303827

[50] Hussain N, Brull R, Sheehy B, Dasu M, Weaver T, Abdallah FW. Does the addition of iPACK to adductor canal block in the presence or absence of periarticular local anesthetic infiltration improve analgesic and functional outcomes following total knee arthroplasty? A systematic review and meta-analysis. Regional Anesthesia and Pain Medicine. 2021;**46**(8):713-721. DOI: 10.1136/rapm-2021-102705

[51] Martin R, Kirkham KR, Ngo THN, Gonvers E, Lambert J, Albrecht E. Combination of femoral triangle block and infiltration between the popliteal artery and the capsule of the posterior knee (iPACK) versus local infiltration analgesia for analgesia after anterior cruciate ligament reconstruction: A randomized controlled triple-blinded trial. Regional Anesthesia and Pain Medicine. 2021;**46**(9):763-768. DOI: 10.1136/rapm-2021-102631

[52] Nguyen KT, Marcelino R, Jagannathan N, Suresh S, Sawardekar A. Infiltration between popliteal artery and capsule of the knee block to augment continuous femoral nerve catheter for adolescent anterior cruciate ligament reconstruction: A case series. A&A Practice. 2020;**14**(2):37-39. DOI: 10.1213/XAA.0000000000001135

[53] Kim D-H, Choi S-S, Yoon S-H, Lee S-H, Seo D-K, Lee I-G, et al. Ultrasound-guided genicular nerve block for knee osteoarthritis: A double-blind, randomized controlled trial of local anesthetic alone or in combination with corticosteroid. Pain Physician. 2018;**21**(1):41-52

[54] Choi W-J, Hwang S-J, Song J-G, Leem J-G, Kang Y-U, Park P-H, et al. Radiofrequency treatment relieves chronic knee osteoarthritis pain: A double-blind randomized controlled trial. Pain. 2011;**152**(3):481-487. DOI: 10.1016/j.pain.2010.09.029

[55] Moradi Tuchayi S, Wang Y, Khodorova A, Pence IJ, Stemmer-Rachamimov A, Evans CL, et al. Fast-acting and injectable cryoneurolysis device. Scientific Reports. 2022;**12**(1):19891. DOI: 10.1038/s41598-022-24178-6

[56] Sunderland S. A classification of peripheral nerve injuries producing loss of function. Brain. 1951;**74**(4):491-516. DOI: 10.1093/brain/74.4.491

[57] Ilfeld BM, Preciado J, Trescot AM. Novel cryoneurolysis device for the treatment of sensory and motor peripheral nerves. Expert Review of Medical Devices. 2016;**13**(8):713-725. DOI: 10.1080/17434440.2016.1204229

[58] Dasa V, Lensing G, Parsons M, Harris J, Volaufova J, Bliss R. Percutaneous freezing of sensory nerves prior to total knee arthroplasty. The Knee. 2016;**23**(3):523-528. DOI: 10.1016/j.knee.2016.01.011

[59] Nygaard N-PB, Koch-Jensen C, Vægter HB, Wedderkopp N, Blichfeldt-Eckhardt M, Gram B. Cryoneurolysis for the management of chronic pain in patients with knee osteoarthritis; a double-blinded randomized controlled sham trial. BMC Musculoskeletal Disorders. 2021;**22**(1):228, 10.1186/s12891-021-04102-1

[60] Tran J, Peng PWH, Lam K, Baig E, Agur AMR, Gofeld M. Anatomical study of the innervation of anterior knee joint capsule: Implication for image-guided intervention. Regional Anesthesia and Pain Medicine. 2018;**43**(4):407-414. DOI: 10.1097/aap.0000000000000778

[61] Ferreira-Dos-Santos G, Hurdle M-FB, Gupta S, Tran J, Agur AMR, Clendenen SR. Revisiting the genicular nerve block: An up-to-date guide utilizing ultrasound guidance and peripheral nerve stimulation - anatomy description and technique standardization. Pain Physician. 2021;**24**(2):E177-E183

[62] Balocco AL, Claes E, Lopez A, Van Herreweghe I. Selective periarticular blocks for postoperative pain after hip and knee arthroplasty. Current Opinion in Anaesthesiology. 2021;**34**(4):544-552. DOI: 10.1097/ACO.0000000000000943

[63] Orduña Valls JM, Vallejo R, López Pais P, Soto E, Torres Rodríguez D, Cedeño DL, et al. Anatomic and ultrasonographic evaluation of the knee sensory innervation: A cadaveric study to determine anatomic targets in the treatment of chronic knee pain. Regional Anesthesia and Pain Medicine. 2017;**42**(1):90-98. DOI: 10.1097/aap.0000000000000516

[64] Ilfeld BM. Continuous peripheral nerve blocks: An update of the published evidence and comparison with novel, alternative analgesic modalities. Anesthesia and Analgesia. 2017;**124**(1):308-335. DOI: 10.1213/ANE.0000000000001581

[65] Zhou L, Kambin P, Casey KF, Bonner FJ, O'Brien E, Shao Z, et al. Mechanism research of cryoanalgesia. Neurological Research. 1995;**17**(4):307-311.DOI:10.1080/01616412.1995.11740333

[66] Kerns JM, Braverman B, Mathew A, Lucchinetti C, Ivankovich AD. A comparison of cryoprobe and crush lesions in the rat sciatic nerve. Pain. 1991;**47**(1):31-39. DOI: 10.1016/0304-3959(91)90008-L

[67] Ilfeld BM, Gabriel RA, Trescot AM. Ultrasound-guided percutaneous cryoneurolysis for treatment of acute pain: Could cryoanalgesia replace continuous peripheral nerve blocks? British Journal of Anaesthesia. 2017; **119**(4):709-712. DOI: 10.1093/bja/aex142

[68] Biel E, Aroke EN, Maye J, Zhang SJ. The applications of cryoneurolysis for acute and chronic pain management. Pain Practice. 2023;**23**(2):204-215. DOI: 10.1111/papr.13182

[69] Radnovich R, Scott D, Patel AT, Olson R, Dasa V, Segal N, et al. Cryoneurolysis to treat the pain and symptoms of knee osteoarthritis: A multicenter, randomized, double-blind, sham-controlled trial. Osteoarthritis and Cartilage. 2017;**25**(8):1247-1256. DOI: 10.1016/j.joca.2017.03.006

[70] Trescot AM. Cryoanalgesia in interventional pain management. Pain Physician. 2003;**6**(3):345-360

[71] Akesen S, Akesen B, Atıcı T, Gurbet A, Ermutlu C, Özyalçın A. Comparison of efficacy between the genicular nerve block and the popliteal artery and the capsule of the

posterior knee (IPACK) block for total knee replacement surgery: A prospective randomized controlled study. Acta Orthopaedica et Traumatologica Turcica. 2021;**55**(2):134-140. DOI: 10.5152/j.aott.2021.20187

[72] Layera S, Aliste J, Bravo D, Saadawi M, Salinas FV, Tran DQ. Motor-sparing nerve blocks for total knee replacement: A scoping review. Journal of Clinical Anesthesia. 2021;**68**(110076):110076. DOI: 10.1016/j.jclinane.2020.110076

[73] Said ET, Marsh-Armstrong BP, Fischer SJ, Suresh PJ, Swisher MW, Trescot AM, et al. Relative effects of various factors on ice ball formation and ablation zone size during ultrasound-guided percutaneous cryoneurolysis: A laboratory investigation to inform clinical practice and future research. Pain and Therapy. 2023;**12**(3):771-783. DOI: 10.1007/s40122-023-00497-y

[74] Erskine RN, White L. A review of the external oblique intercostal plane block - a novel approach to analgesia for upper abdominal surgery. Journal of Clinical Anesthesia. 2022;**82**(110953):110953. DOI: 10.1016/j.jclinane.2022.110953

[75] Elsharkawy H, Kolli S, Soliman LM, Seif J, Drake RL, Mariano ER, et al. The external oblique intercostal block: Anatomic evaluation and case series. Pain Medicine. 2021;**22**(11):2436-2442. DOI: 10.1093/pm/pnab296

[76] Schlenz I, Burggasser G, Kuzbari R, Eichberger H, Gruber H, Holle Tulgar J, et al. Perichondral approach for blockage of thoracoabdominal nerves: Anatomical basis and clinical experience in three cases. Journal of Clinical Anesthesia. 1999;**255**(4):8-10

[77] Coşarcan SK, Erçelen Ö. The analgesic contribution of external oblique intercostal block: Case reports of 3 different surgeries and 3 spectacular effects. Medicine (Baltimore). 2022;**101**(36):e30435. DOI: 10.1097/MD.0000000000030435

[78] Coşarcan SK, Yavuz Y, Doğan AT, Erçelen Ö. Can postoperative pain be prevented in bariatric surgery? Efficacy and usability of fascial plane blocks: A retrospective clinical study. Obesity Surgery. 2022;**32**(9):2921-2929. DOI: 10.1007/s11695-022-06184-9

[79] Liotiri D, Diamantis A, Papapetrou E, Grapsidi V, Sioka E, Stamatiou G, et al. External oblique intercostal (EOI) block for enhanced recovery after liver surgery: A case series. Anaesthesia Reports. 2023;**11**(1):e12225. DOI: 10.1002/anr3.12225

[80] Nielsen KC, Guller U, Steele SM, Klein SM, Greengrass RA, Pietrobon R. Influence of obesity on surgical regional anesthesia in the ambulatory setting: An analysis of 9,038 blocks. Anesthesiology. 2005;**102**(1):181-187. DOI:10.1097/00000542-200501000-00027

[81] White L, Ji A. External oblique intercostal plane block for upper abdominal surgery: Use in obese patients. British Journal of Anaesthesia. 2022;**128**(5):e295-e297. DOI: 10.1016/j.bja.2022.02.011

[82] Tulgar S, Senturk O, Selvi O, Balaban O, Ahiskalioğlu A, Thomas DT, et al. Perichondral approach for blockage of thoracoabdominal nerves: Anatomical basis and clinical experience in three cases. Journal of Clinical Anesthesia. 2019;**54**:8-10. DOI: 10.1016/j.jclinane.2018.10.015

[83] U.S. Food and Drug Administration, Center for Drug Evaluation and Research. EXPAREL NDA 022496 Approval letter. 2013 October 28.

2011. Available from: http://www.accessdata.fda.gov/drugsatfda_docs/appletter/2011/022496s000ltr.pdf [Accessed: May 2023]

[84] Saraghi M, Hersh EV. Three newly approved analgesics: An update. Anesthesia Progress. 2013;**60**(4):178, 10.2344/0003-3006-60.4.178-187

[85] Jin Z, Ding O, Islam A, Li R, Lin J. Comparison of liposomal bupivacaine and conventional local anesthetic agents in regional Anesthesia: A systematic review. Anesthesia and Analgesia. 2021;**132**(6):1626-1634. DOI: 10.1213/ANE.0000000000005406

[86] Bergese SD, Ramamoorthy S, Patou G, Bramlett K, Gorfine SR, Candiotti KA. Efficacy profile of liposome bupivacaine, a novel formulation of bupivacaine for postsurgical analgesia. Journal of Pain Research. 2012;**5**:107-116. DOI: 10.2147/JPR.S30861

[87] Ilfeld BM, Eisenach JC, Gabriel RA. Clinical effectiveness of liposomal bupivacaine administration by infiltration or peripheral nerve block to treat postoperative pain. Anesthesiology. 2021;**134**(2):283-344. DOI: 10.1097/ALN.0000000000003630

[88] Davidovitch R, Goch A, Driesman A, Konda S, Pean C, Egol K. The use of liposomal bupivacaine administered with standard bupivacaine in ankle fractures requiring open reduction internal fixation: A single-blinded randomized controlled trial. Journal of Orthopaedic Trauma. 2017;**31**:434-439. DOI: 10.1097/BOT.0000000000000862

[89] Higgins JP, Altman DG, Gøtzsche PC, Jüni P, Moher D, Oxman AD, et al. Cochrane bias methods group; Cochrane statistical methods group: The Cochrane Collaboration's tool for assessing risk of bias in randomized trials. BMJ. 2011;**343**:d5928. DOI: 10.1136/bmj.d5928

[90] Mont MA, Beaver WB, Dysart SH, Barrington JW, Del Gaizo DJ. Local infiltration analgesia with liposomal bupivacaine improves pain scores and reduces opioid use after total knee arthroplasty: Results of a randomized controlled trial. The Journal of Arthroplasty. 2018;**33**:90-96. DOI: 10.1016/j.arth.2017.07.024

[91] Snyder MA, Scheuerman CM, Gregg JL, Ruhnke CJ, Eten K. Improving total knee arthroplasty perioperative pain management using a periarticular injection with bupivacaine liposomal suspension. Arthroplasty Today. 2016;**2**:37-42. DOI: 10.1016/j.artd.2015.05.005

[92] Namdari S, Nicholson T, Abboud J, Lazarus M, Steinberg D, Williams G. Interscalene block with and without intraoperative local infiltration with liposomal bupivacaine in shoulder arthroplasty: A randomized controlled trial. The Journal of Bone and Joint Surgery. American Volume. 2018;**100**:1373-1378. DOI: 10.2106/JBJS.17.01416

[93] Johnson RL, Amundson AW, Abdel MP, Sviggum HP, Mabry TM, Mantilla CB, et al. Continuous posterior lumbar plexus nerve block versus periarticular injection with ropivacaine or liposomal bupivacaine for total hip arthroplasty: A three-arm randomized clinical trial. The Journal of Bone and Joint Surgery. American Volume. 2017;**99**:1836-1845. DOI: 10.2106/JBJS.16.01305

[94] Amundson AW, Johnson RL, Abdel MP, Mantilla CB, Panchamia JK, Taunton MJ, et al. A three arm randomized clinical trial comparing continuous femoral plus single-injection

sciatic peripheral nerve blocks *versus* periarticular injection with ropivacaine or liposomal bupivacaine for patients undergoing total knee arthroplasty. Anesthesiology. 2017;**126**:1139-1150. DOI: 10.1097/ALN.0000000000001586

[95] Okoroha KR, Keller RA, Marshall NE, Jung EK, Mehran N, Owashi E, et al. Liposomal bupivacaine *versus* femoral nerve block for pain control after anterior cruciate ligament reconstruction: A prospective randomized trial. Arthroscopy. 2016;**32**:838-845. DOI: 10.1016/j.arthro.2016.05.033

[96] Okoroha KR, Lynch JR, Keller RA, Korona J, Amato C, Rill B, et al. Liposomal bupivacaine versus interscalene nerve block for pain control after shoulder arthroplasty: A prospective randomized trial. Journal of Shoulder and Elbow Surgery. 2016;**25**:1742-1748. DOI: 10.1016/j.jse.2016.05.007

[97] Surdam JW, Licini DJ, Baynes NT, Arce BR. The use of Exparel (liposomal bupivacaine) to manage postoperative pain in unilateral total knee arthroplasty patients. The Journal of Arthroplasty. 2015;**30**:325-329. DOI: 10.1016/j.arth.2014.09.004

[98] Talmo CT, Kent SE, Fredette AN, Anderson MC, Hassan MK, Mattingly DA. Prospective randomized trial comparing femoral nerve block with intraoperative local anesthetic injection of liposomal bupivacaine in total knee arthroplasty. The Journal of Arthroplasty. 2018;**33**:3474-3478. DOI: 10.1016/j.arth.2018.07.018

[99] Abildgaard JT, Lonergan KT, Tolan SJ, Kissenberth MJ, Hawkins RJ, Washburn R 3rd, et al. Liposomal bupivacaine *versus* indwelling interscalene nerve block for postoperative pain control in shoulder arthroplasty: A prospective randomized controlled trial. Journal of Shoulder and Elbow Surgery. 2017;**26**:1175-1181. DOI: 10.1016/j.jse.2017.03.012

[100] Marino J, Scuderi G, Dowling O, Farquhar R, Freycinet B, Overdyk F. Periarticular knee injection with liposomal bupivacaine and continuous femoral nerve block for postoperative pain management after total knee arthroplasty: A randomized controlled trial. The Journal of Arthroplasty. 2019;**34**:495-500. DOI: 10.1016/j.arth.2018.11.025

[101] Gasanova I, Alexander J, Ogunnaike B, Hamid C, Rogers D, Minhajuddin A, et al. Transversus abdominis plane block *versus* surgical site infiltration for pain management after open total abdominal hysterectomy. Anesthesia and Analgesia. 2015;**121**:1383-1388. DOI: 10.1213/ANE.0000000000000909

[102] McGraw-Tatum MA, Groover MT, George NE, Urse JS, Heh V. A prospective, randomized trial comparing liposomal bupivacaine vs fascia iliaca compartment block for postoperative pain control in total hip arthroplasty. The Journal of Arthroplasty. 2017;**32**:2181-2185. DOI: 10.1016/j.arth.2017.02.019

[103] Ayad S, Babazade R, Elsharkawy H, Nadar V, Lokhande C, Makarova N, et al. Comparison of transversus abdominis plane infiltration with liposomal bupivacaine versus continuous epidural analgesia versus intravenous opioid analgesia. PLoS One. 2016;**11**(4):e0153675. DOI: 10.1371/journal.pone.0153675.e0153675

[104] Bourn T, Serpa SM. Bupivacaine/meloxicam ER. A new dual-acting extended-release local Anesthetic for opioid-sparing postoperative

pain management. The Annals of Pharmacotherapy. 2023;**57**(1):71-85. DOI: 10.1177/10600280221086639

[105] Soto G, González MN, Calero F. Intravenous lidocaine infusion. Revista Española de Anestesiología y Reanimación (English Edition). 2018;**65**(5):269-274. DOI: 10.1016/j.redar.2018.01.004

[106] Weibel S, Jelting Y, Pace NL, Helf A, Eberhart LH, Hahnenkamp K, et al. Continuous intravenous perioperative lidocaine infusion for postoperative pain and recovery in adults. Cochrane Database of Systematic Reviews. 2018;**6**(6):CD009642. DOI: 10.1002/14651858.CD009642.pub3

[107] Tan H, Wan T, Guo W, Fan G, Xie Y. Mepivacaine versus bupivacaine for spinal anesthesia: A systematic review and meta-analysis of randomized controlled trials. Advances in Therapy. 2022;**39**(5):2151-2164. DOI: 10.1007/s12325-022-02088-3

[108] Siddiqi A, Mahmoud Y, Secic M, Tozzi JM, Emara A, Piuzzi NS, et al. Mepivacaine versus bupivacaine spinal anesthesia for primary total joint arthroplasty: A systematic review and meta-analysis. Journal of Arthroplasty. 2022;**37**(7):1396-1404.e5. DOI: 10.1016/j.arth.2022.03.031

[109] Fu Z, Tang X, Wang D, Liu L, Li J, Chen J, et al. Mepivacaine versus bupivacaine in adult surgical patients: A meta-analysis, trial sequential analysis of randomized controlled trials. Journal of Perianesthesia Nursing. 2022;**37**(6):872-882.e1. DOI: 10.1016/j.jopan.2022.01.011

[110] Shah J, Votta-Velis EG, Borgeat A. New local anesthetics. Best Practice & Research. Clinical Anaesthesiology. 2018;**32**(2):179-185. DOI: 10.1016/j.bpa.2018.06.010

[111] Boublik J, Gupta R, Bhar S, Atchabahian A. Prilocaine spinal anesthesia for ambulatory surgery: A review of the available studies. Anaesthesia, Critical Care & Pain Medicine. 2016;**35**(6):417-421. DOI: 10.1016/j.accpm.2016.03.005

[112] Carvalho B, Sultan P. Spinal prilocaine for caesarean section: Walking a fine line. Anaesthesia. 2021;**76**(6):740-742. DOI: 10.1111/anae.15341

[113] Zhang Y, Yang J, Yin Q, Yang L, Liu J, Zhang W. QX-OH, a QX-314 derivative agent, produces long-acting local anesthesia in rats. European Journal of Pharmaceutical Sciences. 2017;**105**:212-218. DOI: 10.1016/j.ejps.2017.05.039

[114] Yin Q, Zhang Y, Lv R, Gong D, Ke B, Yang J, et al. A fixed-dose combination, QXOH/levobupivacaine, produces long-acting local anesthesia in rats without additional toxicity. Frontiers in Pharmacology. 2019;**10**:243. DOI: 10.3389/fphar.2019.00243

[115] Zhang Y, Yin Q, Gong D, Kang Y, Yang J, Liu J, et al. The preclinical pharmacological study of a novel long-acting local anesthetic, a fixed-dose combination of QX-OH/levobupivacaine, in rats. Frontiers in Pharmacology. 2019;**10**:895. DOI: 10.3389/fphar.2019.00895

[116] Zhang J, Zhang Y, Yin Q, Yang J, Kang Y, Gong D, et al. The 14-day repeated-dose toxicity study of a fixed-dose combination, QXOH/levobupivacaine, via subcutaneous injection in beagle dogs. Journal of Applied Toxicology. 2021;**41**(8):1241-1261. DOI: 10.1002/jat.4111

[117] Yang Y, Wang C, Liu J, Liao D, Zhang W, Zhou C. QX-OH/levobupivacaine: A structurally novel, potent local Anesthetic produces

fast-onset and long-lasting regional Anesthesia in rats. Journal of Pain Research. 2022;**15**:331-340. DOI: 10.2147/JPR.S343500

[118] Zhang W, Xu W, Ning C, Li M, Zhao G, Jiang W, et al. Long-acting hydrogel/microsphere composite sequentially releases dexmedetomine and bupivacaine for prolonged synergistic analgesia. Biomaterials. 2018;**181**:378-391. DOI: 10.1016/j.biomaterials.2018.07.051

[119] Chen S, Yao W, Wang H, Wang T, Xiao X, Sun G, et al. Injectable electrospun fiber-hydrogel composite sequentially releasing clonidine and ropivacaine for prolonged and walking regional anesthesia. Theranostics. 2022;**12**(11):4904-4921. DOI: 10.7150/thno.74845

[120] Desai N, Albrecht E, El-Boghdadly K. Perineural adjuncts for peripheral nerve block. BJA Education. 2019;**19**(9):276-282. DOI: 10.1016/j.bjae.2019.05.001

[121] Chan AKM, Cheung CW, Chong YK. Alpha-2 agonists in acute pain management. Expert Opinion on Pharmacotherapy. 2010;**11**(17):2849-2868. DOI: 10.1517/14656566.2010.511613

[122] Weerink MAS, Struys MMRF, HannivoortLN,BarendsCRM,AbsalomAR, Colin P. Clinical pharmacokinetics and pharmacodynamics of dexmedetomidine. Clinical Pharmacokinetics. 2017;**56**(8):893-913. DOI: 10.1007/s40262-017-0507-7

[123] Ranganath Y, Seering M, Marian A. Curb your enthusiasm: Local anesthetic adjuvants for peripheral nerve blocks. ASRA News. 2020;**45**(4). Available from: https://www.asra.com/news-publications/asra-newsletter/newsletter-item/asra-news/2020/11/01/curb-your-enthusiasm-local-anesthetic-adjuvants-for-peripheral-nerve-blocks

[124] Tang C, Xia Z. Dexmedetomidine in perioperative acute pain management: A non-opioid adjuvant analgesic. Journal of Pain Research. 2017;**10**:1899-1904. DOI: 10.2147/JPR.S139387

[125] Vorobeichik L, Brull R, Abdallah FW. Evidence basis for using perineural dexmedetomidine to enhance the quality of brachial plexus nerve blocks: A systematic review and meta-analysis of randomized controlled trials. British Journal of Anaesthesia. 2017;**118**:167-181

[126] Choi S, Rodseth R, McCartney CJL. Effects of dexamethasone as a local anaesthetic adjuvant for brachial plexus block: A systematic review and meta-analysis of randomized trials. British Journal of Anaesthesia. 2014;**112**(3):427-439. DOI: 10.1093/bja/aet417

[127] Bei T, Liu J, Huang Q, Wu J, Zhao J. Perineural versus intravenous dexamethasone for brachial plexus block: A systematic review and meta-analysis of randomized controlled trials. Pain Physician. 2021;**24**(6):E693-E707. Available from: https://www.painphysicianjournal.com/current/pdf?article=NzMwOQ%3D%3D&journal=138.y

[128] Pehora C, Pearson AM, Kaushal A, Crawford MW, Johnston B. Dexamethasone as an adjuvant to peripheral nerve block. Cochrane Database of Systematic Reviews. 2017;**11**:CD011770. DOI: 10.1002/14651858.CD011770.pub2

[129] Desai N, Kirkham KR. Albrecht local anaesthetic adjuncts for peripheral regional anaesthesia: A narrative review. Anaesthesia. 2021;**76**(S1):100-109. DOI: 10.1111/anae.15245

[130] Oliveira D, Almeida GS, Benzon MD. McCarthy perioperative single dose systemic dexamethasone

for postoperative pain. Anesthesiology. 2011;**115**(3):575-588. DOI: 10.1097/aln.0b013e31822a24c2

[131] Bravo D, Aliste J, Layera S, Fernández D, Leurcharusmee P, Samerchua A, et al. A multicenter, randomized comparison between 2, 5, and 8 mg of perineural dexamethasone for ultrasound-guided infraclavicular block. Regional Anesthesia and Pain Medicine. 2019;**44**(1):46-51. DOI: 10.1136/rapm-2018-000032

Chapter 4

Complications in Spinal Anesthesia

Javier Aquiles Hidalgo Acosta, Freddy Octavio Zambrano Hidalgo, María Fernanda Calderón León and Johnny Jerez Castañeda

Abstract

The justification of this chapter is based on knowing the neurological complications that can be triggered during or after spinal anesthesia since it is one of the most performed procedures in anesthesiology, the main objective is to make a chapter with the most described complications in spinal anesthesia. What are the complications of spinal anesthesia? What complications have been described during the procedure or during its postoperative recovery? The spinal anesthesia technique is a necessary procedure to perform a surgical intervention whose objective is to temporarily block the brain's ability to recognize painful stimuli. Knowing possible complications that can occur during spinal anesthesia or in the postoperative period allows for early diagnosis and treatment. Complications in anesthesia can be clinically manifested by headache, gluteal pain that radiates to the lower limbs, neuropathy, severe paresthesia, among others, and can generate reversible and irreversible disabling lesions depending on their mechanism of injury.

Keywords: complications, adverse effects, mortality, spinal anesthesia, care postoperative

1. Introduction

The theme addressed is of great importance for the field of anesthesiology; spinal anesthesia is an invasive technique necessary for regional blockages and is one of the most carried out in surgical interventions, so that recognizing the pathophysiology of neurological damage, diagnosing and treating the complications that may occur the question that starts this chapter What are the neurological complications of spinal anesthesia?

Spinal anesthesia is a technique widely used for its efficacy and safety, and it is also known as spinal, subarachnoid, intradural, or intrathecal anesthesia. It is characterized by the administration of an anesthetic in the subarachnoid space that is located between the pia mater and arachnoid meninges in order to generate a sequential block in the nerve fibers. The neurological complications of spinal anesthesia are of great importance in anesthesiology because some can be serious and be due to multiple previous patients, pharmacological, and genetic factors that can intervene in the complications, as it is a technique widely used in surgery and anesthesiology. When it is necessary to perform a surgical intervention whose objective is to interrupt the connection between the peripheral nervous system and the brain, spinal anesthesia is used to block painful stimuli. This technique and its complications recognize them and immediately treat the complications that occur during or after the anesthetic act [1].

Nerve injury related to the block is a disabling complication of spinal anesthesia, usually seen during the surgical procedure, postoperatively, and some patients may require an intensive care unit. This technique is a procedure used for interventions on the lower extremities, hip, perineum, lower abdomen, and lumbar spine [2].

2. Pathophysiology of neurological complications

Physiopathologically, there are multiple complications of neurological origin that can arise after spinal anesthesia. To do this, we must know the three mechanisms by which a peripheral nerve can suffer an injury [3].

- Mechanical or traumatic injury
- Vascular or ischemic injury
- Chemical or neurotoxic injury

The mechanical injury of the nerve can be due to contact between the needle and the nerve [4], causing direct trauma to the nerve, rupture of the perineurium, loss of the protective environment within the fascicle with myelin, and consequent axonal degeneration. The location of the needle tip during anesthetic injection plays a crucial role in the severity of nerve injury; needlestick injuries during puncture can cause nerve injury by several mechanisms [5].

Damage to the nerve vasculature during blocks can cause local or diffuse ischemia from direct injury or acute occlusion of the arteries or from hemorrhage within a nerve sheath [6].

Local anesthetics and adjuncts reduce neural blood flow depending on the agent and their concentration, for example, epinephrine reduces neural blood flow to a greater extent than local anesthetics alone and has the potential to cause local vasoconstriction [7].

Chemical nerve injury results from tissue toxicity of injected solutions (e.g., local anesthetics, alcohol, or phenol) or their additives. The toxic solution can be injected directly into the nerve or into adjacent tissues, causing an acute inflammatory reaction or chronic fibrosis involving the nerve [8].

The neurotoxicity of local anesthetics has been done in in vitro models, particularly with intrathecal application. There is evidence that almost all local anesthetics can have myotoxic, neurotoxic, and cytotoxic effects in various tissues under certain conditions; however, local anesthetics vary in their neurotoxic potential [9].

In mechanisms of neurological damage, the main determinant of the prognosis is the residual integrity of the axons, and the severity of the lesion is classified according to the degree of axonal interruption in neuropraxia, axonotmesis, and neurotmesis [10].

Among the factors that influence neurological injury are surgical factors [11].

2.1 Surgical positioning

Neurological complications occur as a result of patient positioning for surgical procedures (**Figures 1** and **2**), and these include traction, transection, compression, contusion, ischemia, and stretch [12]. Nerve roots are more susceptible to traction and compression because they lack epineural and perineural tissue; however, the dorsal and

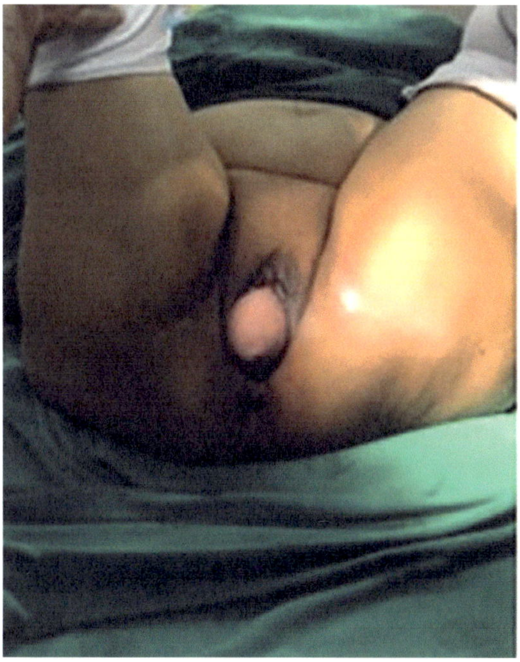

Figure 1.
Description: Lithotomy position. Source: Dr. María Fernanda Calderón León.

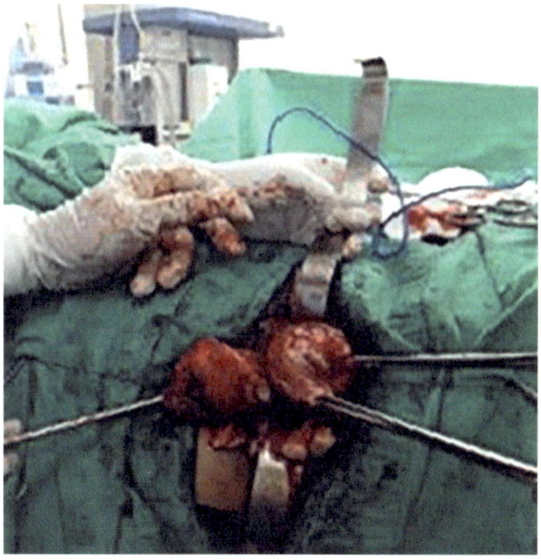

Figure 2.
Description: Transvaginal hysterectomy surgical procedure plus anterior and posterior colpoperioneoraphy, a procedure that lasts about 2 to 4 hours, keeping the patient in the same position. Source: Dr. María Fernanda Calderón León.

ventral roots of the spinal nerves are protected from lateral traction by the wedge of a cone of dura mater that surrounds the spinal-root nerve complex at the intervertebral foramen [13].

A history of preoperative neurologic deficit places a patient at increased risk of neuronal injury and can result from several mechanisms: entrapment, metabolic, ischemic, toxic, and demyelinating. Patients with preexisting pathology of the spinal canal have a higher incidence of neurological complications after neuraxial blockade than patients without such pathology. Lumbar disc injuries increase the risk of neurological complications of spinal anesthesia [14, 15].

3. Types of neurological complications of spinal anesthesia

- Postspinal puncture headache is the most common complication of spinal anesthesia and may be accompanied by chest pain, neck pain, and depression. Management includes early recognition, admission for analgesic management, and neuroimaging studies to rule out other pathologies [16, 17].

- Pneumocephalus is characterized by postsurgical neurological signs such as headache, neck stiffness, altered level of consciousness, or respiratory depression in the most severe cases [18].

- Cauda equina syndrome as a complication may occur and is characterized by bilateral weakness and pain in the lower extremities after the anesthetic act. This may indicate transient or persistent neurological damage due to involvement of the cauda equina of the spinal cord, and it may be asymmetric with a unilateral deficit and present after neuraxial anesthesia, which may complicate the postoperative period and require additional studies such as electromyography, tomography, or magnetic resonance imaging and multidisciplinary management [19–21].

- Hypotension during the intraoperative phase of spinal anesthesia may complicate preexisting coronary artery disease, worsen prior mental decline, or precipitate stroke [22].

- A reversible pathology is the transient neurological syndrome that is clinically manifested by gluteal pain that radiates to the lower limbs, neuropathy, and severe paresthesia is transient with recovery after neurorehabilitation, patients recover functionality [23].

- Spinal hematomas account for 8% of neuraxial anesthesia complications. Subdural hematoma, epidural hematoma, may require surgical management, after which symptoms can resolve [24].

- Cerebral venous thrombosis and cerebral ischemia comprise two catastrophic complications; cases of this complication following spinal anesthesia have been described and generate high mortality [25].

- toxic or infectious encephalomyelitis after spinal anesthesia can cause symptoms characterized by neurological deterioration, facial paralysis, cranial nerve III paralysis, paraplegia, and cerebral edema in diagnostic studies such as brain tomography [26].

- The cases of myelitis, myelinolysis (**Figure 3**), are infrequent; they are observed in the immediate postoperative period with a new deficit or lack of neurological recovery measured by the anesthetic recovery scales, the spinal cord damage is only observed in the magnetic resonance (MRI) of the spinal cord or altered MRI of the brain in cases of myelinolysis [27].

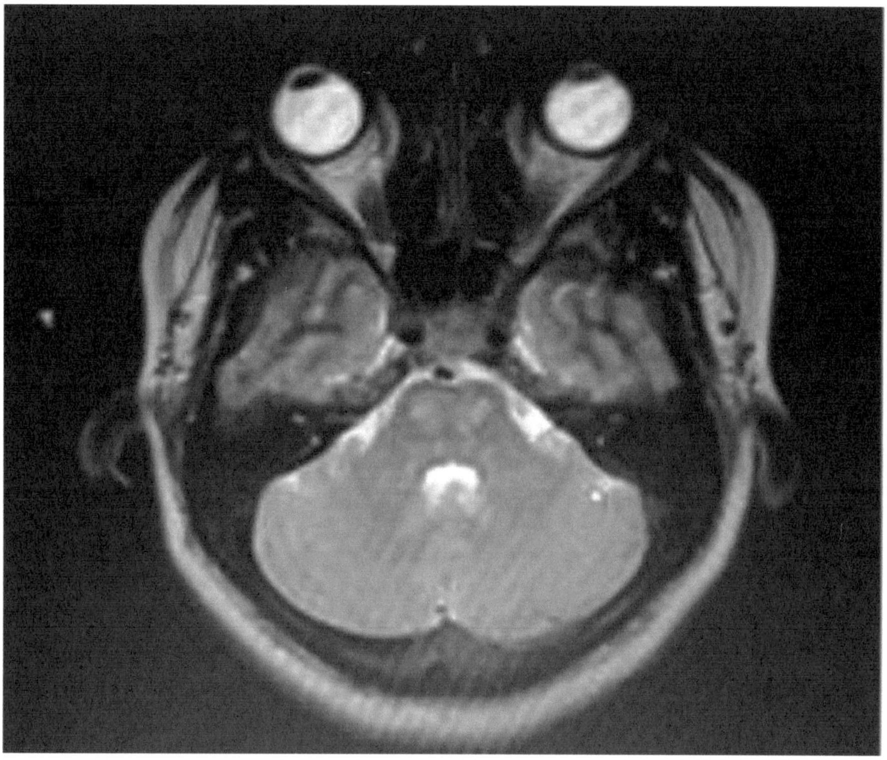

Figure 3.
Source: Javier Aquiles, Hidalgo Acosta. Description: Myelinolysis.

Author	Complication	Management	Recommendation	Diagnosis
Vallejo M, et al	Postdural puncture headache	Nonopioid analgesics, opioids, supine position, Follow-up the first 24–48 h	Spinal needles of "pencil tip" design that do not cut	CT, MRI
Ahmad M, et al.	Pneumocephalus	Analgesia, 40–100% oxygen, supine position	Pneumocephalus requires immediate surgical intervention	CT
Merino W, et al.	Cauda equina syndrome	Pregabalin, tramadol, dexamethasone, methylprednisolone	Early detection and treatment of complications after neuraxial anesthesia	Lumbar MRI
Lacassie H, et al.	Epidural infection, Postmeningeal puncture Meningitis	Antibiotic therapy for *Staphylococci* sp., *Staphylococcus aureus*, *Viridans Streptococcus*, *Pseudomonas aeruginosa*, Alpha-hemolytic *Streptococci*	Use sterile cap, mask, and gloves, and perform skin asepsis with chlorhexidine prior	Lumbar puncture and study of cerebrospinal fluid

Author	Complication	Management	Recommendation	Diagnosis
Freire F, et al	Cauda equina Syndrome	Corticosteroids, gastric mucosa protectors and rehabilitation, carbamazepine, and amitriptyline	Perform a thorough history and complete evaluation to rule out external causes	Axial tomography computerized lumbosacral spine Column nuclear magnetic Resonance lumbosacral, motor sensory conduction velocity in lower limbs
Hewson D, et al.	Peripheral nerve injury	Objectives: 1. correct the underlying pathology; 2. alleviate the symptoms; 3. support, reassure and inform the patient	Nerve localization methods, the timing of blocks, needle techniques and design, injection pressure control, and choice of local and adjunctive anesthetic	Further investigation of possible causes of nerve injury should be conducted by a neurologist and neurophysiologist
Epstein N	Intracranial hypotension, subdural hematomas, and double vision/ cranial nerve palsy	Clinical – surgical	Detect potential neurological risks/ complications/ adverse events	MRI of the brain, spine, CT of the brain and spine
Russell R, et al.	Cerebral vein thrombosis and death	Headache treatment	Adequate follow-up after discharge	CT and MRI of the brain
Arce D, et al.	Toxic encephalomyelitis	Intravenous betamethasone at a rate of 24 mg on the first day, with progressive reduction. The patient was maintained with 8 mg intravenous for 2 months, associated with physiotherapy sessions	Neurorehabilitation, admission to the intensive care unit	Brain CT

Source: Javier Aquiles, Hidalgo Acosta.

Table 1.
Complications of spinal anesthesia, diagnosis, management, and recommendation.

Description: The (**Table 1**) represents complications of spinal anesthesia that can be mild or severe, the diagnosis, treatment, and the recommendations of the authors for the management of complications of spinal anesthesia.

4. Conclusions

This review maintains the intended significance as it provides practical knowledge of the possible complications that may arise during the performance of this invasive spine technique.

Neurological complications in anesthesia can be mild, such as headache, transient a paradigm neurological syndrome is clinically manifested by gluteal pain that radiates to the lower limbs, neuropathy, and severe paresthesia, among others; serious complications can be fatal. It is important to be aware of complications.

The pain reported by the patient when advancing the needle or injecting the medication may indicate the placement of the needle at the intraneural level, so the injection must be stopped.

Patients with preexisting pathology of the spinal canal have a higher incidence of neurological complications after neuraxial blockade than patients without such pathology.

Complications can be due to multiple factors, all of which can be responsible for neurological complications. Blockade-related nerve injury remains one of the most common disabling complications.

Acknowledgements

A special thank you to my mother, teacher Mrs. Juana Narcisa Acosta Alcívar, an example to follow in education in Ecuador, Abigucho, Claris, Lucciana.

This is done with full funding from the authors.

Conflict of interest

The authors declare no conflict of interest.

Notes/thanks/other declarations

Thanks.

Appendices and nomenclature

CT	computed tomography
MRI	Magnetic nuclear resonance

Author details

Javier Aquiles Hidalgo Acosta[1*], Freddy Octavio Zambrano Hidalgo[2], María Fernanda Calderón León[3] and Johnny Jerez Castañeda[4]

1 Teodoro Maldonado Carbo Hospital, Critical Medicine Specialist, Anesthesiology Unit, Guayaquil, Ecuador

2 Higher Polytechnic Agricultural School of Manabí Manuel Félix López, ESPAM MFL University, Manabí, Ecuador

3 Matilde Hidalgo De Procel Hospital, Specialist in Gynecology and Obstetrics, Guayaquil, Ecuador

4 General Hospital of the North of Guayaquil, Ecuador

*Address all correspondence to: jahidalgoacosta@hotmail.com

References

[1] Neuman MD, Feng R, Carson JL, Gaskins LJ, Dillane D, Sessler DI, et al. Regain investigators. Spinal Anesthesia or general Anesthesia for hip surgery in older adults. The New England Journal of Medicine. 2021;**385**(22):2025-2035. DOI: 10.1056/NEJMoa2113514

[2] Rathmell JP, Avidan MS. Patient-centered outcomes after general and spinal anesthesia. The New England Journal of Medicine. 25 Nov 2021;**385**(22):2088-2089. DOI: 10.1056/NEJMe2116017

[3] Waters JFR. Neurological complications of obstetric Anesthesia. Continuum (Minneap Minn). 2022;**28**(1):162-179. DOI: 10.1212/CON.0000000000001073

[4] Althagafi A, Nadi M. Acute nerve injury. In: StatPearls. Treasure Island (FL): StatPearls Publishing; 2022 May 5 [Internet]

[5] Biso GMNR, Munakomi S. Neuroanatomy, Neurapraxia. 2021 Oct 30. In: StatPearls. Treasure Island (FL): StatPearls Publishing; 2022 [Internet]

[6] Pozza DH, Tavares I, Cruz CD, Fonseca S. Spinal cord injury and complications related to neuraxial anaesthesia procedures: A systematic review. International Journal of Molecular Science. 28 Feb 2023;**24**(5):4665. DOI: 10.3390/ijms24054665

[7] Hidalgo Acosta JA, Mawyin Muñoz CE, Cujilema Parreño MC, González Echeverría KE, Montenegro Jara JL, Ruiz Alejandro MR, et al. Anestesia espinal y sus complicaciones neurológicas. Un artículo de revisión de la literatura. MedicienciasUTA [Internet]. 1 de octubre de 2022 [citado 3 de octubre de 2023];**6**(4):9-15. Disponible en: https://revistas.uta.edu.ec/erevista/index.php/medi/article/view/1830

[8] Liu H, Brown M, Sun L, Patel SP, Li J, Cornett EM, et al. Complications and liability related to regional and neuraxial anesthesia. Best Practice & Research. Clinical Anaesthesiology. 2019;**33**(4):487-497. DOI: 10.1016/j.bpa.2019.07.007. Epub 2019 Jul 19

[9] Kent CD, Stephens LS, Posner KL, Domino KB. What adverse events and injuries are cited in Anesthesia malpractice claims for nonspine orthopedic surgery? Clinical Orthopaedics and Related Research. 2017;**475**(12):2941-2951. DOI: 10.1007/s11999-017-5303-z

[10] Huang H, Yao D, Saba R, Brovman EY, Kang D, Greenberg P, et al. A contemporary medicolegal claims analysis of injuries related to neuraxial anesthesia between 2007 and 2016. Journal of Clinical Anesthesia. 2019;**57**:66-71. DOI: 10.1016/j.jclinane.2019.03.013. Epub 2019 Mar 12

[11] Hemmings HC Jr, Riegelhaupt PM, Kelz MB, Solt K, Eckenhoff RG, Orser BA, et al. Toward a comprehensive understanding of anesthetic mechanisms of action: A decade of discovery. Trends in Pharmacological Sciences. Jul 2019;**40**(7):464-481. DOI: 10.1016/j.tips.2019.05.001

[12] Munro C, Baliga S, Shepherd J, MacEachern CF. Anatomical study of the human sacral hiatus and implications for successful caudal epidural injection. The Surgeon. 2021;**19**(5):e103-e106. DOI: 10.1016/j.surge.2020.08.010

[13] Pirenne V, Dewinter G, Van de Velde M. Spinal anaesthesia in obstetrics. Best Practice and Research Clinical

Anaesthesiology. Jun 2023;**37**(2):101-108. DOI: 10.1016/j.bpa.2023.03.006

[14] Saba R, Brovman EY, Kang D, Greenberg P, Kaye AD, Urman RD. A contemporary Medicolegal analysis of injury related to peripheral nerve blocks. Pain Physician. 2019;**22**(4):389-400

[15] Gelb AW, Morriss WW, Johnson W, et al. World Health Organization-world Federation of Societies of Anesthesiologists (WHO-WFSA) international standards for the safe practice of anesthesia. Canadian Journal of Anaesthesia/Journal Canadien D'anesthésie. 2018;**65**:698-708. DOI: 10.1007/s12630-018-1111-5

[16] Vallejo MC, Zakowski MI. Post-dural puncture headache diagnosis and management. Best Practice & Research. Clinical Anaesthesiology. 2022;**36**(1):179-189. DOI: 10.1016/j.bpa.2022.01.002

[17] Mims SC, Tan HS, Sun K, Pham T, Rubright S, Kaplan SJ, et al. Long-term morbidities following unintentional dural puncture in obstetric patients: A systematic review and meta-analysis. Journal of Clinical Anesthesia. 2022;**79**:110787. DOI: 10.1016/j.jclinane.2022.110787

[18] Sotosek V. Changes in mental status and transient bradypnea due to pneumocephalus after the application of epidural anesthesia: A case report. Annals of Clinical and Medical Case Reports. 2019;**2**(4):1-4

[19] Merino-Urrutia W, Villagrán-Schmidt M, Ulloa-Vásquez P, Carrasco-Moyano R, Uribe A, Stoicea N, et al. Cauda equina syndrome following an uneventful spinal anesthesia in a patient undergoing drainage of the Bartholin abscess: A case report. Medicine (Baltimore). 2018;**97**(19):e0693. DOI: 10.1097/MD.0000000000010693

[20] Lacassie HJ, Lacassie M, Lacassie E. Complicaciones neurológicas e infecciones tras analgesia neuroaxial del parto. Revista Chilena de Anestesia. 2022;**51**(6):623-635. DOI: 10.25237/revchilanestv5127091144

[21] Freire Guerra F, Hualpa Freire A, Teran PP. Complication of spinal anesthesia for knee surgery: Cauda Equina syndrome. Mediciencias UTA. [Internet]. 1 Sep 2018;**2**(3):32-36. Available from: https://revistas.uta.edu.ec/erevista/index.php/medi/ar

[22] Vives R, Fernandez-Galinski D, Gordo F, Izquierdo A, Oliva JC, Colilles C, et al. Effects of bupivacaine or levobupivacaine on cerebral oxygenation during spinal anesthesia in elderly patients undergoing orthopedic surgery for hip fracture: a randomized controlled trial. BMC Anesthesiol. 31 Jan 2019;**19**(1):17. DOI: 10.1186/s12871-019-0682-1

[23] Hewson DW, Bedforth NM, Hardman JG. Peripheral nerve injury arising in anaesthesia practice. Anaesthesia. Jan 2018;**73**(Suppl 1):51-60. DOI: 10.1111/anae.14140

[24] Epstein NE. Neurological complications of lumbar and cervical dural punctures with a focus on epidural injections. Surgical Neurology International. 26 Apr 2017;**8**:60. DOI: 10.4103/sni.sni_38_17

[25] Russell R, Laxton C, Lucas DN, Niewiarowski J, Scrutton M, Stocks G. Treatment of obstetric post-dural puncture headache. Part 2: epidural blood patch. International Journal of Obstetric Anesthesia. May 2019;**38**:104-118. DOI: 10.1016/j.ijoa.2018.12.005

[26] Arce PD, Albín CRG. Encefalomielitis tóxica por anestesia espinal. Presentación de un caso. Medisur [Internet]. 2021 Abr [citado 2023 Mayo 12];**19**(2):274-279. Disponible en: http://scielo.sld.cu/scielo.php?script=sci_arttext&pid=S1727-897X2021000200274&lng=es

[27] Urtubia R, Tevah J, Catalán P, et al. Mielitis transversa aguda asociada a anestesia espinal: Caso clínico. Revista Chilena de Anestesia. 2022;**51**(5):602-605. DOI: 10.25237/revchilanestv5106071542

Chapter 5

Regional Anesthesia for Cardiac Surgery

Sarah Smith, Kaya Sarier, Richard Yeom and Ian Choe

Abstract

Cardiac surgery is associated with significant postoperative pain, regardless of surgical approach. Median sternotomy and thoracotomy are particularly traumatic, resulting in pain that typically lasts weeks and may lead to chronic pain syndromes. Even newer minimally invasive procedures involving mini-thoracotomy and other smaller incisions are not pain-free, while the presence of chest tubes also causes significant discomfort. Uncontrolled pain following cardiac surgery contributes to adverse outcomes, particularly pulmonary complications and prolonged lengths of stay. Intravenous opiates alone or in combination with other sedatives are imperfect solutions to this problem as they are associated with excess sedation, nausea, vomiting, pruritis, delirium, constipation, and dependence. In recent years, regional anesthesia techniques have increasingly been utilized for cardiac surgery as part of enhanced recovery after cardiac surgery pathways. In many cases, techniques that were developed for other surgical procedures, particularly breast surgery, have been applied to the cardiac surgical population with favorable results. However, many practicing cardiac anesthesiologists have limited experience with these regional anesthesia techniques, so implementing them into clinical practice effectively can be challenging. This chapter aims to address this gap by reviewing the evidence, techniques, and applicability of the regional anesthesia approaches appropriate for cardiac surgery patients.

Keywords: post-sternotomy pain, post-thoracotomy pain, enhanced recovery after cardiac surgery, regional anesthesia techniques, ultrasound guided nerve blockade

1. Introduction

Effective pain management is crucial in cardiac surgery to optimize patient outcomes and reduce postoperative complications. Cardiac anesthesia has significantly changed over the last 50 years, evolving from earlier techniques that utilized high doses of opiates and other narcotics to a more balanced approach that incorporates the principles of enhanced recovery after cardiac surgery (ERACS). This review aims to provide a comprehensive overview of the regional anesthesia techniques currently in use for cardiac surgeries, including median sternotomy, thoracotomy, and minimally invasive approaches. The relevant anatomy, technique, and pharmacology for each regional technique will be described as well as their clinical applications, complications, and contraindications. The techniques will be described in anatomical order, centrally to peripherally, beginning with neuraxial approaches and ending with the most peripheral parasternal nerve blocks.

2. Neuraxial techniques

Spinal and epidural anesthesia and analgesia techniques involve administering local anesthetics, with or without adjuvant medications, into either the subarachnoid or epidural space, respectively, providing potent sensory, motor, and sympathetic depression in the region of the block. The use of neuraxial techniques in cardiac surgery has been controversial due to the potential for hemodynamic instability and the concern for spinal or epidural hematoma [1]. However, evidence suggests that appropriate use of these techniques has numerous advantages, including improved patient outcomes and healthcare cost savings [2].

2.1 Anatomical considerations

The spinal cord is protected by the cervical (C1-7), thoracic (T1-12), and lumbar vertebrae (L1-5) and is encased by three membranes: the dura, arachnoid, and pia mater. The dura encases the brain, spinal cord, and the spinal nerve roots, which are suspended in cerebrospinal fluid. The location of the caudal end of the spinal cord, or conus medullaris, is somewhat variable between individuals, usually terminating at the level of L1 or L2 in adults and L3 in children. Therefore, spinal anesthesia is usually performed at the level of L3/4 or L4/5 to avoid damage to the spinal cord. Intrathecally injected local anesthetics exert their effects directly on the spinal cord and the emerging spinal roots, providing potent nerve blockade with relatively small doses of local anesthetic [3].

The epidural space surrounds the dura from the foramen magnum to the sacrococcygeal ligament and is defined by the ligamentum flavum posteriorly, the vertebral pedicles laterally, and the posterior longitudinal ligament anteriorly. It contains fat, epidural blood vessels, lymphatics, and the spinal nerve roots. Local anesthetics injected into the epidural space exert their effects at these nerve roots and on the spinal cord itself via diffusion through the dura [4]. For this reason, much larger doses of local anesthetics must be administered to achieve the desired effect compared to intrathecally injected medications. However, this also allows epidural anesthesia to be more easily titrated to a desired level of sensory or motor blockade. Further, because epidural anesthesia does not involve puncture of the dura, there is little risk of direct spinal cord trauma, and the technique can be applied anywhere from the mid-thoracic to the lower lumbar regions [5].

2.2 Epidural anesthesia and analgesia

Thoracic epidural anesthesia has been used to augment general anesthesia and provide postoperative pain control in the cardiac surgery population for more than 20 years. A large meta-analysis of 51 randomized clinical trials found that compared to general anesthesia alone, thoracic epidural anesthesia decreased ICU length of stay (LOS), hospital LOS, and time to extubation. Statistically significant improvements in pain scores, pulmonary complications, arrhythmias, transfusion requirements, and delirium were also identified [6]. Other contemporary meta-analyses have yielded similar findings [7, 8], with one of these also finding a modest decrease in mortality [7].

Recently, neuraxial blockades have been gaining attention in pediatric cardiac surgery [9]. Compared to general anesthesia alone, caudal anesthesia may provide superior pain control [10]. Caudal anesthesia has also been shown to decrease intraoperative opioid usage [11], decrease the time to extubation, and reduce hospital LOS [12]. However, there have been conflicting reports in the literature regarding the potential for hemodynamic instability following caudal anesthesia in pediatric patients undergoing cardiac surgery [10, 13, 14].

2.2.1 Technique

Thoracic epidural catheters may be inserted using either a midline or paramedian approach. In the midline approach, the epidural needle (typically a 17 or 18G Touhy) is inserted into the middle of the patient's back between two spinous processes. The needle is advanced through the supraspinous ligament and interspinous ligament. Once the needle has reached the interspinous ligament, the stylet is removed and a syringe is attached to enable the detection of loss of resistance to air, saline, or both, which represents penetration of the ligamentum flavum and identification of the epidural space.

For the paramedian approach, the epidural needle is introduced 1 centimeter lateral and 1 centimeter caudad to the inferior portion of the superior spinous process. The needle is advanced until the lamina of the vertebral body below is encountered. The needle is then directed 15–20° medially before advancing cephalad such that the needle "walks off" the lamina until the ligamentum flavum is encountered. A loss of resistance technique is then used as in the midline approach.

The paramedian approach may be a better option for patients who cannot flex their spine or when midline approaches are unsuccessful. For the midline approach in the thoracic region, the epidural needle must take a steeply angled trajectory parallel to the direction of the spinous processes. For this reason, some practitioners prefer the paramedian approach for thoracic epidurals [15]. The paramedian approach can also be facilitated by real-time ultrasound guidance [16] and may be associated with less procedure-related back pain compared to the midline approach [17].

The caudal approach to the epidural space is used frequently in pediatrics. The epidural space is accessed through the sacral hiatus, which is a foramen formed by the nonunion of the fifth sacral vertebral body. To perform a caudal block, the patient is positioned either lateral or prone and the sacral hiatus is identified as the apex of an equilateral triangle formed together with the superior inferior iliac spines. The bony processes, called the sacral cornua, on either side can also be palpated to identify the space. The epidural needle is inserted at a 45° angle directed cephalad until a popping sensation is felt as the needle pierces the sacrococcygeal membrane. The needle is then flattened until it is nearly parallel to the plane of the skin and advanced into the sacral canal until loss of resistance is encountered [18].

2.2.2 Complications and contraindications

Any patient with a spinal cord injury, epidural or spinal cord hematoma, intracranial hypertension, or vertebral fracture is not a candidate for neuraxial anesthesia due to a high risk of neurological complications [1]. Patient refusal, bacteremia, and infection at the insertion site of the epidural needle are also absolute contraindications [19]. Patients with coagulopathic disorders such as hemophilia should not receive neuraxial anesthesia due to the increased risk of epidural or spinal hematoma.

Generally, a platelet count of less than 50,000 per microliter or an INR greater than 1.5 is also considered absolute contraindications [1].

Because many cardiac surgery patients are maintained on anti-platelet and other anticoagulant agents, it is important to observe the American Society of Regional Anesthesia and Pain Management guidelines regarding how long these drugs should be discontinued before neuraxial anesthesia and when it is safe for them to be resumed post-procedure [20]. Many cardiac anesthesiologists have been reluctant to incorporate epidural anesthesia into their practice because of a concern that systemic heparinization required for cardiopulmonary bypass increases the risk of epidural hematoma, a devastating complication that can lead to permanent paralysis. The literature is unclear regarding exactly how high this risk is in the cardiac population, with some authors finding that the rate may be as high as 1 in 3552 [7], while others have estimated the value as 1 in 12,000, a rate similar to that observed in the non-obstetric non-cardiac surgery population [21].

2.3 Spinal anesthesia and analgesia

The use of spinal anesthesia in cardiac surgery has been limited, however, authors from one center have reported using bupivacaine and opiates intrathecally to augment general anesthesia in over 10,000 cardiac surgery patients. They also reported no incidents of spinal hematoma and favorable pain control [1]. Another group found intrathecal morphine administered prior to minimally invasive cardiac surgery decreased visual analog pain scores and intravenous opiate usage post-operatively [22]. A meta-analysis of intrathecal morphine compared to general anesthesia alone in cardiac surgical patients also found decreases in pain scores and post-operative opiate use at the expense of increased pruritis [23].

2.3.1 Technique

The intrathecal space may be accessed using either a midline or paramedian approach, as described above for epidural anesthesia. Unlike the epidural technique, a much smaller needle (typically a 25-27G cutting or pencil point needle) is used to deliberately pierce the dura until free-flowing CSF is observed to exit the needle. After this, the desired amount of local anesthetic or adjuvant medication is injected into the subarachnoid space [3].

2.3.2 Complications and contraindications

Contraindications to spinal anesthesia are similar to those for epidural anesthesia, including patient refusal, coagulopathy, neurologic dysfunction, intracranial hypertension, local skin infection, and bacteremia. Unlike epidural anesthesia via a catheter, in which local anesthetic can be introduced gradually into the epidural space, spinal anesthesia requires that these agents be injected as a single shot. This can have more profound and abrupt changes in hemodynamics and may not be tolerated by patients who are dependent on the maintenance of preload or blood pressure, such as those with severe aortic stenosis.

While spinal anesthesia also confers a risk of neurologic damage from hematoma formation, this risk is substantially less than that for epidural anesthesia [24]. Because spinal anesthesia necessitates a puncture of the dura, there is also a risk for post-dural puncture headache of up to 25%, however, the incidence in the cardiac surgical population is not well established.

3. Posterior thoracic wall blocks

The thoracic paravertebral plane block (PVB) and erector spinae plane block (ESPB) with or without catheter placement have emerged as potential options for providing effective analgesia following cardiac surgery, particularly those performed via thoracotomy such as thoracic aneurysm repair, mitral valve procedures, and minimally invasive cardiac surgery procedures.

3.1 Anatomical considerations

The PVB involves the injection of local anesthetic into the paravertebral space (PVS), which is located just anterior to the transverse process and lateral to the vertebral bodies. It is a triangular space bounded by the superior costotransverse ligament, the vertebral body, and the pleura. This space contains the paravertebral sympathetic chain, intercostal nerve roots, and associated blood vessels (**Figure 1**). The block targets the spinal nerves as they emerge from the intervertebral foramina before they split into the ventral and dorsal rami, as well as the thoracic sympathetic nerves which mediate visceral pain. This makes the PVB more complete compared with other chest wall blocks with an area of analgesic distribution that makes it appropriate for a variety of thoracic procedures, including sternotomy. Just posterior to the paravertebral space is the retro-superior costotransverse space (RSCTS). This is bounded by the superior costotransverse ligament, the transverse process and the erector spinal muscle. There are communications between the RSCTS and the PVS, so injectate administered in the RSCTS will reach the PVS as well [25].

The ESPB, on the other hand, involves injection of local anesthetic into the erector spinae muscle plane which is located lateral to the transverse process of the vertebrae. The local anesthetic spreads along this fascial plane, acting on the dorsal and ventral rami, blocking the posterior and lateral cutaneous intercostal nerves. Some of the

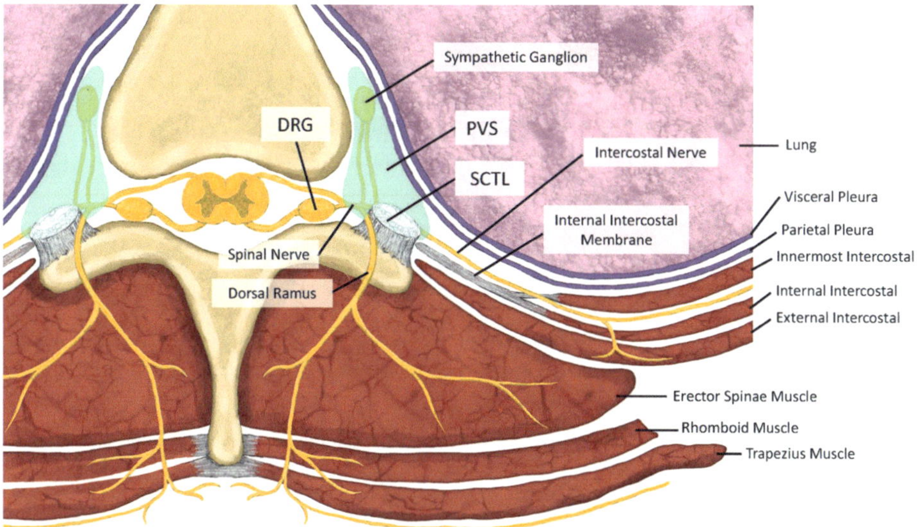

Figure 1.
The anatomy of the paravertebral space (green). PVS: paravertebral space; SCTL: superior costotransverse ligament; and DRG: dorsal root ganglion.

injectates may penetrate the paravertebral space, potentially blocking multiple levels of spinal nerves, although not as densely as the PVB. While a T2-10 block is possible with the ESPB, the distribution is highly variable in clinical practice [26].

3.2 Paravertebral block

Unilateral PVB has been shown to improve patient outcomes for a variety of thoracic procedures, including thoracic aneurysm repair. Bilateral PVB for sternotomy has also been shown to decrease the time to extubation and the need for intra- and post-operative intravenous opiates in both adults and children [27].

3.2.1 Technique

The PVB is typically performed at the level of the surgical incision or one or two vertebral levels above and below the surgical site, depending on the dermatomal distribution of the surgical field. Although originally described using a loss of resistance technique [28], real-time ultrasound guidance has now become the standard approach. The anatomy is best visualized using a linear or curvilinear ultrasound probe in the parasagittal orientation 2.5 cm lateral to the spinous process (**Figure 2**). The block may be performed with the patient in a sitting, lateral, or prone position. The injection is usually performed in-plane, and the needle may be directed either cranially or caudally [29].

The PVB can also be performed with the ultrasound probe in the transverse orientation, and the PVS identified by identifying the transverse process and then scanning either cranially or caudally [30]. One cadaveric study found this approach was slightly less successful than the parasaggital approach [31]. With either technique, the needle should be placed anterior to the superior costotransverse ligament, and a 3 mL test dose administered demonstrating anterior displacement of the pleura [29]. The dosage of local anesthetic for a single injection is 20–25 mL or 4–5 mL per level, and for catheter placement, a continuous infusion of local anesthetic at 0.1–0.2 mL/kg/h is often used [32].

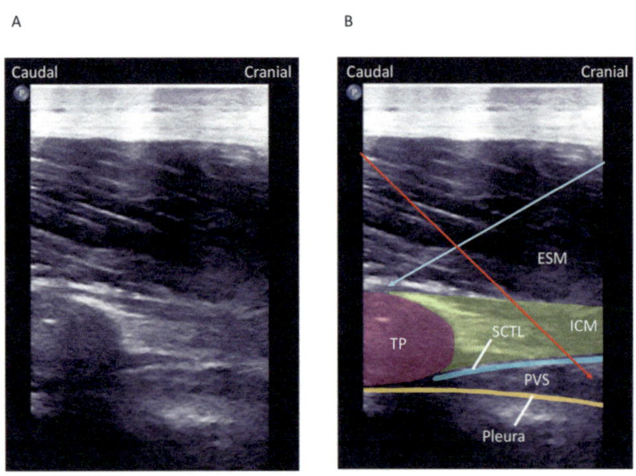

Figure 2.
(A) Ultrasound image for ESPB or PVB. (B) Labeled ultrasound image showing proper needle trajectory and injection site for the ESPB (blue arrow) and PVB (red arrow). ESM: erector spinae muscle; TP: transverse process; SCTL: superior costotransverse ligament; PVS: paravertebral space; and ICM: intercostal muscle.

3.2.2 Complications and contraindications

Because of the proximity to the spine, rare complications of the PVB can include epidural or spinal hematoma or infection. If a catheter is placed, this is more likely if the catheter is advanced more than 3–4 cm beyond the needle tip. Pneumothorax is also possible, and the risk is minimized with proper use of ultrasound. More common reactions include hemodynamic instability due to sympathetic blockade, which is more likely to occur after a bolus of more concentrated preparations of local anesthetic. The overall risk of adverse effects is roughly 5% [33]. However, a recent meta-nalysis of PVB compared to thoracic epidural for open thoracotomy, found that while analgesia was similar between the two techniques, PVB was associated with less nausea, vomiting, urinary retention, and hypotension [34].

3.3 Erector spinae plane block

The ESPB can be used either as a single-shot or continuous catheter-based technique for either preemptive or rescue analgesia for patients undergoing thoracotomy or other thoracic surgery. Some studies, including those on cardiac surgery patients, have found equal analgesic benefits when compared to PVB, but with a lower risk of hypotension, bradycardia, and hematoma [35, 36].

3.3.1 Technique

The ESPB is typically performed at the level of the surgical site or one or two vertebral levels above or below the surgical field, depending on the spread of the local anesthetic needed. The ultrasound probe should be oriented in the parasagittal plane approximately 2.5 cm lateral to the spinous process similar to probe placement for the PVB (**Figure 2**). It may be possible to identify the three overlying muscle layers: the trapezius, rhomboid, and erector spinae. The needle should be directed in-plane either cranially or caudally with injectate directed just deep to the erector spinae muscles. If correctly placed, the injectate should demonstrate lifting of the erector spinae muscle off transverse process [37].

3.3.2 Complications and contraindications

The risk of complications with the ESPB is thought to be low, but pneumothorax, and motor blockade, have been reported [38–40]. Like the PVB, there is a rare but potential risk of neurologic complications, including epidural or spinal hematoma. However, this risk is less than with PVB because of the more lateral point of needle insertion away from the spinal cord. Sympathetic blockade may also be observed resulting in hypotension. While either the PVB or the ESPB can be expected to cover 4 dermatomes if 30 ml of local anesthetic is used, the distribution and degree of coverage are more variable and less complete with the ESPB.

4. Lateral chest wall blocks

The lateral chest wall blocks are relatively new techniques, only coming into use within the last decade. Although ineffective in providing analgesia for median sternotomy, these blocks can be useful for procedures involving incisions of the lateral chest, including thoracotomies and newer minimally invasive approaches to coronary bypass [41]. The pectoralis nerve block type I (PECS I), pectoralis nerve block type II (PECS II), and serratus anterior plane block (SAP) all achieve analgesia by blocking the intercostal and pectoral nerves at different points along the chest wall [42–44].

4.1 Anatomical considerations

The sensory innervation of the anterior and lateral chest wall is mainly carried by the intercostal nerves (T1–T11). After exiting the vertebral foramen, each thoracic spinal nerve travels anteriorly via ventral rami. Initially, the ventral rami travels between the innermost intercostal muscle and the internal intercostal muscle. As the intercostal nerve reaches the midaxillary line, the lateral cutaneous branch crosses the intercostal and serratus anterior muscles, providing sensory innervation to the lateral chest wall. The rest of intercostal nerve continues to course toward the sternum and pierces the internal and external intercostal muscles as well as the pectoralis major muscle, providing sensory innervation to the anterior chest wall via the anterior branch [45]. The sensory innervation to the lateral chest wall is also supplied by the branches of the brachial plexus, most notably the lateral pectoral nerve [46].

4.2 Pectoralis nerve block type I and II

The PECS I block was first described by Blanco in 2011 as an effective postoperative analgesia block for patients undergoing breast surgery [42]. It is an interfascial plane block in which local anesthetic is injected between the pectoralis major and pectoralis minor at the level of the third rib [45]. The PECS I aims to block the medial and lateral pectoral nerves which are branches of the brachial plexus. These two nerves mostly provide motor innervation; however, the lateral pectoral nerve also provides sensory innervation to the anterolateral chest wall. The distribution of analgesic coverage provided by PECS I depends on the location of the injection of local anesthetic. If injected more medially, the local anesthetic can spread toward the midline, providing anterior chest wall coverage by blocking the anterior intercostal nerve branches [47].

The PECS II block, introduced a year after PECS I, targets a deeper fascial plane between the pectoralis minor and serratus anterior, blocking the anterior divisions of the thoracic intercostal nerves from T2–T6, the long thoracic nerve, and the thoracodorsal nerve [43]. The coverage of the anterior cutaneous intercostal nerves provides more anterior chest wall coverage compared to PECS I [48]. As a result, PECS II is rarely performed in isolation and is instead used in addition to PECS I such that analgesic coverage is provided to the anterior and lateral portions of the chest wall.

The PECS I and II blocks are used widely for patients undergoing breast surgery and there is a limited body of evidence supporting their use in thoracotomies and video-assisted thoracic surgeries, often in combination with the SAP block [49]. One randomized controlled trial (RCT) of 100 adult patients undergoing cardiac surgery via thoracotomy demonstrated the superiority of both the PECS II and SAP blocks compared to intercostal nerve blocks in terms of reduced need for fentanyl rescue and improved visual analog scale (VAS) scores at 8, 10, and 12 hours [50]. These investigators also reported similar findings in a pediatric population undergoing thoracotomy for cardiac surgery [51]. There are also reports of the PECS II block being used either alone or in combination with general anesthesia for cardiac device implantation and transcatheter cardiac procedures [49]. While several groups have reported using

PECS I and II blocks either alone [52] or in combination with parasternal blocks [53] for post-sternotomy analgesia, there is only one RCT of 40 adult patients showing superior analgesia and decreased opioid requirements compared to patients receiving systemic opioids [48].

4.2.1 Technique

The PECS I and II blocks are performed under ultrasound guidance. The patient is positioned supine with the ipsilateral arm either beside the chest or abducted at a 90° angle. With the probe in the parasagittal plane, the subclavian vessels are identified along with the second rib. The probe is then moved inferiorly to the level of the third rib where the pectoralis major and minor muscles are identified. Once the pane between the pectoralis major and minor is identified, the needle is inserted into the plane using an in-plane technique, and the local anesthetic is injected at the interfascial plane between the two muscles [42].

When performing both blocks, PECS II is usually performed first with the injection of local anesthetics between pectoralis minor and serratus anterior (**Figure 3**). The needle is, then, withdrawn to the fascial plane between pectoralis major and pectoralis minor for PECS I block [43].

4.2.2 Complications and contraindications

PECS I & II are considered very safe blocks with the very low rate of complications. Possible complications associated with PECS I & II include injury to the thoracoacromial artery, hematoma, infection, pneumothorax, intravascular injection, and local anesthetic systemic toxicity (LAST) [41].

4.3 Serratus anterior nerve plane block

The SAP block was the third chest wall fascial block described by Blanco and colleagues in 2013. In comparison to PECS II, SAP block has more inferolateral level of

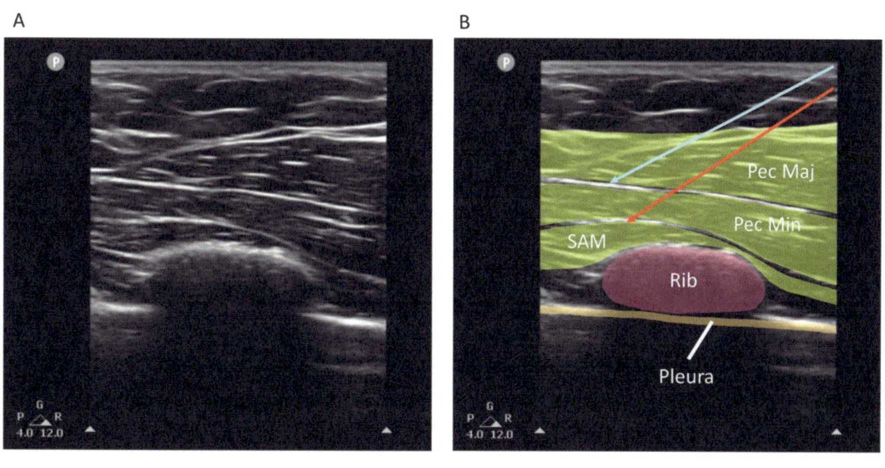

Figure 3.
(A) Ultrasound image for PECS I and II block. (B) Labeled ultrasound image showing proper needle trajectory and injection site for the PEC I (blue arrow) and PEC II (red arrow). SAM: serratus anterior muscle; Pec Maj: pectoralis major muscle; and Pec Min: pectoralis minor muscle.

injection and has a wider spread, which makes it a popular choice for patients undergoing breast surgery or thoracic surgeries. The SAP block provides coverage of the anterior, lateral, and posterior chest wall; however, it does not extend to the midline and is, therefore, inappropriate for median sternotomy [44].

Although the lack of anterior chest wall coverage limits its use for cardiac surgery with sternotomy, SAP block has a potential role in postoperative analgesia in cardiac surgery patients undergoing thoracotomy incisions. Currently, there is no study of SAP block on patients undergoing median sternotomy; however, given the wide use of SAP block for video-assisted thoracoscopic surgery, SAP block may have a role in patients undergoing minimally invasive cardiac surgeries that require mini thoracotomy incisions [49]. One limiting factor is that mini-thoracotomy incisions for minimally invasive cardiac surgery are usually located at the anterolateral chest, which may not be adequately covered by the SAP block alone. In this case, based on the expected coverage, PECS II block may be required to supplement the SAP block. Likewise, if SAP block is used for patients undergoing sternotomy, it is recommended that SAP be performed along with transversus thoracic muscle plane (TTP) or PECS II block [54].

4.3.1 Technique

There are two fascial targets for SAP: superficial and deep. For the superficial SAP, the local anesthetic is injected at the fascial plane between Latissimus dorsi muscle and serratus anterior muscle. For the deep SAP block, the local anesthetic is injected below the serratus anterior muscle (**Figure 4**). It is unclear whether one technique is better than the other; however, it has been suggested that deep SAP may have a more anterior spread of local anesthetic, thereby providing slightly more anterior coverage [44].

As with all plane blocks, the spread is dependent on the volume of local anesthetics. It is recommended that 30–40 mL of long-acting local anesthetic be injected for adequate spread while staying under the maximum limit to prevent LAST [41].

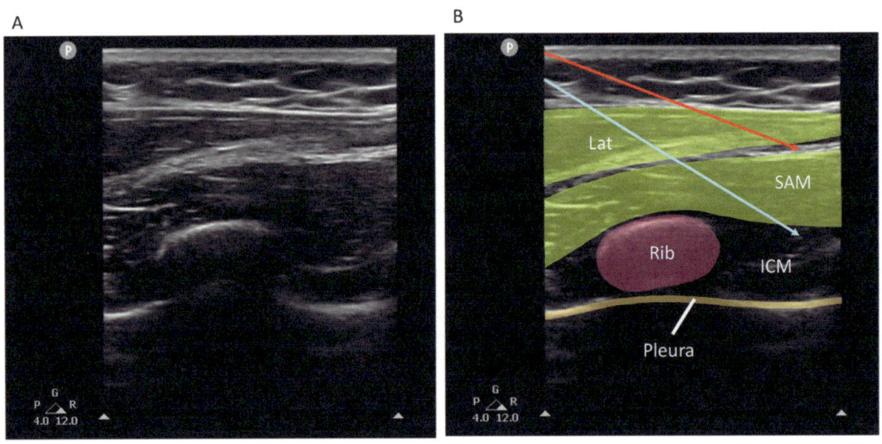

Figure 4.
(A) Ultrasound image for SAP block. (B) Labeled ultrasound image showing proper needle trajectory and injection site for the deep SAP block (blue arrow) and superficial SAP block (red arrow). SAM: serratus anterior muscle; Lat: latissimus dorsi muscle; and ICM: intercostal muscle.

4.3.2 Complications and contraindications

Like PECS I & II, SAP block also has a very low rate of complication. Potential complications of SAP are similar to the complications of PECS I & II, with an additional risk of winging of scapula from the blockade of long thoracic nerve for superficial SAP as the long thoracic nerve runs on top of the serratus anterior muscle [41].

5. Parasternal blocks

Parasternal blocks are emerging techniques that can provide targeted pain relief in the anterior thoracic wall, which is commonly incised during cardiac surgery. Among the various parasternal blocks, pecto-intercostal fascial plane block (PIFB) and transversus thoracic plane block (TTP) are commonly used for postoperative pain management following median sternotomy [55]. Additionally, the subcostal transverse abdominal plane block can be used for subxiphoid chest tube coverage in cardiac surgery. Both the PIFB and the TTP can be used as part of a multimodal analgesic approach in cardiac surgery to provide effective pain relief and reduce the need for systemic opioids. They are relatively simple to perform, provide effective analgesia and have a low risk of adverse effects. Subsequently, the European Society of Regional Anesthesia and Pain Therapy recently added parasternal blocks to their recommendations for managing post-sternotomy pain [56]. These blocks can be performed preoperatively, intraoperatively, or postoperatively and they can be used in combination with other regional anesthesia techniques, such as thoracic epidural analgesia or paravertebral block, to achieve optimal pain control.

5.1 Anatomical considerations

To understand the parasternal blocks, it is important to review the relevant anatomy. The thoracic wall is composed of intercostal muscles, nerves, blood vessels, and fascial planes. The intercostal nerves originate from the anterior rami of the thoracic spinal nerves and course around the lateral chest wall between the internal and innermost internal costal muscles. As the intercostal nerves approach the sternum, they lie between the transversus thoracic muscle and the internal intercostal muscle before piercing the external intercostal membrane as the anterior cutaneous branch [41]. This same facial plane also contains the internal mammary artery and vein which run on either side of the sternum. It is important to identify and avoid these structures when performing parasternal blocks [57]. The anterior cutaneous branch subsequently gives rise to a medial and lateral branch, providing sensory innervation of the skin, subcutaneous tissue, and periosteum of the sternum [41].

5.2 Pecto-intercostal fascial block

The PIFB, also known as pectoral nerve block or pectoral fascial plane block, involves injecting local anesthetic into the plane between the pectoralis major muscle and the intercostal muscles [58, 59]. This is a superficial block, that aims for a T2–T6 sensory blockade of the anterior cutaneous nerve as it makes it way anteriorly. The PIFB is commonly used for pain management in surgeries involving median sternotomy, such as coronary artery bypass grafting (CABG) or valve surgery. The PIFB has been shown to reduce postoperative intravenous opiate consumption, improve pain scores and may decrease the time to extubation following sternotomy [55, 59, 60]. One recent randomized controlled trial compared the TTP to the PIFB and found that they were equivalent in analgesic effectiveness [61].

5.2.1 Technique

Using the ultrasound probe in the parasagittal orientation immediately lateral to the sternum, the rib above and below the desired site of injection are identified. The needle is directed cephalad at an angle of approximately 45° relative to the skin. A popping sensation is often appreciable when the needle enters the facial plane between the pectoralis major muscle and the intercostal muscle. Some practitioners advocate aiming for the inferior surface of the superior rib and then backing the needle back slightly to access the space (**Figure 3**). A test injection of saline should result in an expansion of the space between the two muscle groups. Relatively large volumes of local anesthetic, such as 0.25% bupivacaine or 0.2% ropivacaine, are typically used (20–30 mL per side) to achieve a successful field block. The volume injected can be administered at one site or divided among different intercostal levels which may provide a better spread of local anesthetic [41, 57].

5.2.2 Complications and contraindications

The PIFB is considered a very safe block with a low rate of serious complications. However, care must be taken to avoid inadvertent puncture of the pleura or the pericardium with the block needle. Generally, the PIFB is considered lower risk compared to the TTP block as the facial plane targeted is more superficial and further from the pleura and pericardium [61, 62]. Sterile technique should be fastidiously maintained to avoid infection, particularly in the setting of sternotomy as this could contribute to sternal wound infections. However, a recent meta-analysis of 18 studies evaluating parasternal blocks found no difference in the rate of sternal wound infections compared to control [55]. Appropriate dosing of local anesthetic based on patient weight is also important given the high volumes utilized to avoid LAST [63].

5.3 Transversus thoracic plane block

The transversus thoracic plane (TTP) block is another parasternal block technique that targets the neurovascular plane between the intercostal muscles and the transversus thoracic muscle. The transversus thoracic muscle is very thin and often difficult to distinguish on ultrasound, such that the target area for the block usually appears as a potential space immediately above the pleura. The TTP block is used for postoperative pain management following median sternotomy.

5.3.1 Technique

The ultrasound is oriented in the parasagittal plane at a point somewhat more lateral to the sternum than for the PIFB, typically between the fourth and fifth ribs. The block needle is advanced in-plane at a steeper angle than that utilized for the PIFB until the needle tip traverses the intercostal muscle and enters the space (**Figure 5**). It is important to identify and avoid the internal mammary artery and vein. Local anesthetic dosing is like the PIFB and should be injected slowly under visualization with periodic aspiration to avoid intravascular injection.

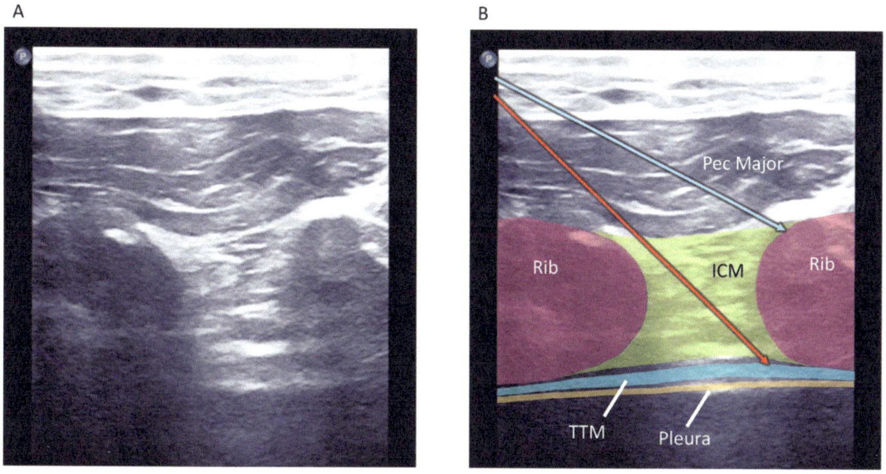

Figure 5.
(A) Ultrasound image for PIFB or TTP block. (B) Labeled ultrasound image showing proper needle trajectory and injection site for the PIFB (blue arrow) and TTP block (red arrow). ICM: intercostal muscle; and TTM: transverse thoracic muscle.

5.3.2 Complications and contraindications

Because the TTP block is deeper than the PIFB, there is a greater risk of puncturing the pleura or pericardium with the block needle. It is important to visualize the internal mammary artery in the long axis to avoid inadvertent puncture of this vessel or unintended arterial injection. The technique is contraindicated following internal mammary artery harvest for coronary bypass surgery as the transversus thoracic muscle is deroofed and the injected local anesthetic will spill into the pleural space [57].

5.4 Transverse abdominal plane block

The transverse abdominal plane (TAP) block has gained popularity in recent years as a component of post-operative multimodal analgesia for abdominal surgeries. When performed in the subcostal region, the TAP block can provide coverage for the subxiphoid chest tube insertion sites typically used for cardiac surgery. The TAP block in this setting is typically used to augment other regional techniques, such as the PIFB and TTP that do not adequately cover chest tube insertion sites. The TAP block involves the injection of local anesthetic between the internal oblique and transverse abdominus muscle and blocks the anterior cutaneous nerves of the T6–T9 dermatome.

5.4.1 Technique

The ultrasound is positioned in the transverse plane immediately caudal to the costal margin on the anterior axillary line. The needle is inserted medial to the probe and is advanced laterally in plane through the rectus abdominus or the linea semilunaris until the space between the transverse abdominus and internal oblique is accessed. Like most other plane blocks, typically large volumes of local anesthetics are used for the subcostal TAP block to achieve adequate distribution. It is important select concentrations and dosages of local anesthetics that do not exceed established safety limits as the subcostal TAP block for cardiac surgery is usually performed in conjunction with the PIFB or TTP block.

5.4.2 Complications and contraindications

TAP blocks have been used widely for approximately 20 years and have an excellent safety record. Inadvertent puncture of abdominal viscera is possible but occurs infrequently if ultrasound guidance is used appropriately. Avoidance of LAST through careful consideration of drug dosages and concentrations is important if the block is performed in conjunction with other regional anesthesia techniques.

6. Conclusion

While the approaches to cardiac surgery were once limited to median sternotomy and thoracotomy, recently surgeons have expanded the use of minimally invasive and percutaneous approaches. However, cardiac surgery continues to be associated with significant postoperative pain which if left uncontrolled can be an impediment to patient recovery. The shortcomings of opiates in mitigating postoperative pain in cardiac surgery patients are many, and anesthesiologists are increasingly utilizing regional anesthesia techniques to reduce the use of these drugs. This review has described the major regional anesthesia techniques being implemented in cardiac surgery patients today, including the contemporary evidence supporting their use.

There is no "one-size-fits-all" approach to regional anesthesia in the cardiac patient, and the specific technique or techniques utilized should depend on the site of the surgical incision, patient factors, and the technical repertoire of the anesthesiologist in question. Institutional factors should also be considered. For example, implementing catheter-based techniques would be unwise if there is not a multidisciplinary team in place to manage the catheters postoperatively. Similarly, integrating regional anesthesia techniques into clinical workflow can be challenging, and should consider the institutional resources available. While some centers rely on cardiac anesthesiologists performing these blocks themselves in the operating room, others have found utilization of a "block team" and pre-operative or post-operative timing of the regional anesthesia procedure to be the most efficient option. Regardless of logistical hurdles, integrating regional anesthesia into the care of cardiac surgical patients has the potential to improve patient outcomes and achieve cost savings for the hospital by reducing length of stay and postoperative complications.

Conflict of interest

The authors declare no conflicts of interest.

Author details

Sarah Smith[1*], Kaya Sarier[1], Richard Yeom[1] and Ian Choe[2]

1 Westchester Medical Center, Valhalla, New York, USA

2 New York Medical College, Valhalla, New York, USA

*Address all correspondence to: scs9006@gmail.com; sarah.smith@wmchealth.org

References

[1] Kowalewski R, Seal D, Tang T, Prusinkiewicz C, Ha D. Neuraxial anesthesia for cardiac surgery: Thoracic epidural and high spinal anesthesia – Why is it different? HSR Proceedings of Intensive Care Cardiovascilar Anesthesia. 2011;**3**(1):25-28

[2] Bignami E, Landoni G, Biondi-Zoccai GG, Boroli F, Messina M, Dedola E, et al. Epidural analgesia improves outcome in cardiac surgery: A meta-analysis of randomized controlled trials. Journal of Cardiothoracic and Vascular Anesthesia. 2010;**24**(4):586-597

[3] Olawin AM. Spinal Anesthesia. Treasure Island, FL: StatPearls; 2023

[4] Avila Hernandez AN, Singh P. Epidural Anesthesia. Treasure Island, FL: StatPearls; 2023

[5] Hermanns H, Bos EME, van Zuylen ML, Hollmann MW, Stevens MF. The options for neuraxial drug administration. CNS Drugs. 2022;**36**(8):877-896

[6] Chiew JK, Low CJW, Zeng K, Goh ZJ, Ling RR, Chen Y, et al. Thoracic epidural anesthesia in cardiac surgery: A systematic review, meta-analysis, and trial sequential analysis of randomized controlled trials. Anesthesia and Analgesia. 1 Sep 2023;**137**(3):587-600

[7] Landoni G, Isella F, Greco M, Zangrillo A, Royse CF. Benefits and risks of epidural analgesia in cardiac surgery. British Journal of Anaesthesia. 2015;**115**(1):25-32

[8] Guay J, Kopp S. Epidural analgesia for adults undergoing cardiac surgery with or without cardiopulmonary bypass. Cochrane Database of Systematic Reviews. 2019;**3**(3):CD006715

[9] Peterson KL, DeCampli WM, Pike NA, Robbins RC, Reitz BA. A report of two hundred twenty cases of regional anesthesia in pediatric cardiac surgery. Anesthesia and Analgesia. 2000;**90**(5):1014-1019

[10] Samantaray DJ, Trehan M, Chowdhry V, Reedy S. Comparison of hemodynamic response and postoperative pain score between general anaesthesia with intravenous analgesia versus general anesthesia with caudal analgesia in pediatric patients undergoing open-heart surgery. Annals of Cardiac Anaesthesia. 2019;**22**(1):35-40

[11] Nguyen KN, Byrd HS, Tan JM. Caudal analgesia and cardiothoracic surgery: A look at postoperative pain scores in a pediatric population. Paediatric Anaesthesia. 2016;**26**(11):1060-1063

[12] Beamer S, Ferns S, Edwards L, Gunther G, Nelson J. Early extubation in pediatric heart surgery across a spectrum of case complexity: Impact on hospital length of stay and chest tube days. Progress in Pediatric Cardiology. 2017;**45**:63-68

[13] Dalens B, Hasnaoui A. Caudal anesthesia in pediatric surgery: Success rate and adverse effects in 750 consecutive patients. Anesthesia and Analgesia. 1989;**68**(2):83-89

[14] Hammer GB, Ngo K, Macario A. A retrospective examination of regional plus general anesthesia in children undergoing open heart surgery. Anesthesia and Analgesia. 2000;**90**(5):1020-1024

[15] McLeod G, Cumming C. Thoracic epidural anaesthesia and analgesia.

Continuing Education in Anaesthesia Critical Care & Pain. 2004;**4**(1):16-19

[16] Pak DJ, Gulati A. Real-time ultrasound-assisted thoracic epidural placement: A feasibility study of a novel technique. Regional Anesthesia and Pain Medicine. 2018;**43**(6):613-615

[17] Hong JH, Cho EY, Shim JW, Park KB. Comparison of postoperative back pain between paramedian and midline approach for thoracic epidural anesthesia. Anesthesia Pain Medicine (Seoul). 2022;**17**(3):320-326

[18] Wiegele M, Marhofer P, Lonnqvist PA. Caudal epidural blocks in paediatric patients: A review and practical considerations. British Journal of Anaesthesia. 2019;**122**(4):509-517

[19] Gerheuser F, Roth A. Epidural anesthesia. Der Anaesthesist. 2007;**56**(5):499-523; quiz 4-6

[20] Horlocker TT, Vandermeuelen E, Kopp SL, Gogarten W, Leffert LR, Benzon HT. Regional anesthesia in the patient receiving antithrombotic or thrombolytic therapy: American Society of Regional Anesthesia and Pain Medicine Evidence-Based Guidelines (Fourth Edition). Regional Anesthesia and Pain Medicine. 2018;**43**(3):263-309

[21] Bracco D, Hemmerling T. Epidural analgesia in cardiac surgery: An updated risk assessment. The Heart Surgery Forum. 2007;**10**(4):E334-E337

[22] Dhawan R, Daubenspeck D, Wroblewski KE, Harrison JH, McCrorey M, Balkhy HH, et al. Intrathecal morphine for analgesia in minimally invasive cardiac surgery: A randomized, placebo-controlled, double-blinded clinical trial. Anesthesiology. 2021;**135**(5):864-876

[23] Chen IW, Sun CK, Ko CC, Fu PH, Teng IC, Liu WC, et al. Analgesic efficacy and risk of low-to-medium dose intrathecal morphine in patients undergoing cardiac surgery: An updated meta-analysis. Frontier in Medicine (Lausanne). 2022;**9**:1017676

[24] Moen V, Dahlgren N, Irestedt L. Severe neurological complications after central neuraxial blockades in Sweden 1990-1999. Anesthesiology. 2004;**101**(4):950-959

[25] Karmakar MK. Thoracic paravertebral block. Anesthesiology. 2001;**95**(3):771-780

[26] Marshall K, McLaughlin K. Pain management in thoracic surgery. Thoracic Surgery Clinics. 2020;**30**(3):339-346

[27] Sahajanandan R, Varsha AV, Kumar DS, Kuppusamy B, Karuppiah S, Shukla V, et al. Efficacy of paravertebral block in "fast-tracking" pediatric cardiac surgery – Experiences from a tertiary care center. Annals of Cardiac Anaesthesia. 2021;**24**(1):24-29

[28] Eason MJ, Wyatt R. Paravertebral thoracic block-a reappraisal. Anaesthesia. 1979;**34**(7):638-642

[29] D'Ercole F, Arora H, Kumar PA. Paravertebral block for thoracic surgery. Journal of Cardiothoracic and Vascular Anesthesia. 2018;**32**(2):915-927

[30] Krediet AC, Moayeri N, van Geffen GJ, Bruhn J, Renes S, Bigeleisen PE, et al. Different approaches to ultrasound-guided thoracic paravertebral block: An illustrated review. Anesthesiology. 2015;**123**(2):459-474

[31] Ruscio L, Renard R, Lebacle C, Zetlaoui P, Benhamou D, Bessede T. Thoracic paravertebral block: Comparison of different approaches and techniques. A study on 27 human cadavers.

Anesthesia Critical Care Pain Medicine. 2020;**39**(1):53-58

[32] Nair S, Gallagher H, Conlon N. Paravertebral blocks and novel alternatives. BJA Education. 2020;**20**(5):158-165

[33] Ardon AE, Lee J, Franco CD, Riutort KT, Greengrass RA. Paravertebral block: Anatomy and relevant safety issues. Korean Journal of Anesthesiology. 2020;**73**(5):394-400

[34] Ren P, Du Y, He G, Jiang D. Efficacy and safety of general anesthesia combined with paravertebral blockade on postoperative recovery in patients undergoing pulmonary surgery: A systematic review and meta-analysis. Journal of Thoracic Disease. 2022;**14**(2):431-442

[35] Adhikary SD, Prasad A, Soleimani B, Chin KJ. Continuous erector spinae plane block as an effective analgesic option in anticoagulated patients after left ventricular assist device implantation: A case series. Journal of Cardiothoracic and Vascular Anesthesia. 2019;**33**(4):1063-1067

[36] Fang B, Wang Z, Huang X. Ultrasound-guided preoperative single-dose erector spinae plane block provides comparable analgesia to thoracic paravertebral block following thoracotomy: A single center randomized controlled double-blind study. Annals of Translational Medicine. 2019;**7**(8):174

[37] Kot P, Rodriguez P, Granell M, Cano B, Rovira L, Morales J, et al. The erector spinae plane block: A narrative review. Korean Journal of Anesthesiology. 2019;**72**(3):209-220

[38] De Cassai A, Geraldini F, Carere A, Sergi M, Munari M. Complications rate estimation after thoracic erector spinae plane block. Journal of Cardiothoracic and Vascular Anesthesia. 2021;**35**(10):3142-3143

[39] De Cassai A, Fasolo A, Geraldini F, Munari M. Motor block following bilateral ESP block. Journal of Clinical Anesthesia. 2020;**60**:23

[40] Hamilton DL. Pneumothorax following erector spinae plane block. Journal of Clinical Anesthesia. 2019;**52**:17

[41] Kelava M, Alfirevic A, Bustamante S, Hargrave J, Marciniak D. Regional anesthesia in cardiac surgery: An overview of fascial plane chest wall blocks. Anesthesia and Analgesia. 2020;**131**(1):127-135

[42] Blanco R. The 'pecs block': A novel technique for providing analgesia after breast surgery. Anaesthesia. 2011;**66**(9):847-848

[43] Blanco R, Fajardo M, Parras MT. Ultrasound description of Pecs II (modified Pecs I): A novel approach to breast surgery. Revista Española de Anestesiología y Reanimación. 2012;**59**(9):470-475

[44] Blanco R, Parras T, McDonnell JG, Prats-Galino A. Serratus plane block: A novel ultrasound-guided thoracic wall nerve block. Anaesthesia. 2013;**68**(11):1107-1113

[45] Pectoralis and Serratus Plane Nerve Blocks. Available from: https://www.nysora.com/topics/regional-anesthesia-for-specific-surgical-procedures/thorax/pectoralis-serratus-plane-blocks/

[46] Desroches J, Belliveau M, Bilodeau C, Landry M, Roy M, Beaulieu P. Pectoral nerves I block is associated with a significant motor blockade with no dermatomal sensory changes: A prospective volunteer

randomized-controlled double-blind study. Canadian Journal of Anaesthesia. 2018;**65**(7):806-812

[47] Versyck B, Groen G, van Geffen GJ, Van Houwe P, Bleys RL. The pecs anesthetic blockade: A correlation between magnetic resonance imaging, ultrasound imaging, reconstructed cross-sectional anatomy and cross-sectional histology. Clinical Anatomy. 2019;**32**(3):421-429

[48] Kumar KN, Kalyane RN, Singh NG, Nagaraja PS, Krishna M, Babu B, et al. Efficacy of bilateral pectoralis nerve block for ultrafast tracking and postoperative pain management in cardiac surgery. Annals of Cardiac Anaesthesia. 2018;**21**(3):333-338

[49] Jack JM, McLellan E, Versyck B, Englesakis MF, Chin KJ. The role of serratus anterior plane and pectoral nerves blocks in cardiac surgery, thoracic surgery and trauma: A qualitative systematic review. Anaesthesia. 2020;**75**(10):1372-1385

[50] Magoon R, Kaushal B, Chauhan S, Bhoi D, Bisoi AK, Khan MA. A randomised controlled comparison of serratus anterior plane, pectoral nerves and intercostal nerve block for post-thoracotomy analgesia in adult cardiac surgery. Indian Journal of Anaesthesia. 2020;**64**(12):1018-1024

[51] Kaushal B, Chauhan S, Saini K, Bhoi D, Bisoi AK, Sangdup T, et al. Comparison of the efficacy of ultrasound-guided serratus anterior plane block, pectoral nerves II block, and intercostal nerve block for the management of postoperative thoracotomy pain after pediatric cardiac surgery. Journal of Cardiothoracic and Vascular Anesthesia. 2019;**33**(2):418-425

[52] Freedman Z, AuBuchon J, Montana M. A single-center descriptive account of the use of pectoral nerve I and II nerve blocks for post-operative pain relief following pediatric sternotomy. Paediatric Neonatal Pain. 2023;**5**(1):16-22

[53] Ata F, Yilmaz C. Retrospective evaluation of fascial plane blocks in cardiac surgery with median sternotomy in a tertiary hospital. Cureus. 2023;**15**(3):e35718

[54] Ritter MJ, Christensen JM, Yalamuri SM. Regional Anesthesia for cardiac surgery: A review of fascial plane blocks and their uses. Advances in Anesthesia. 2021;**39**:215-240

[55] King M, Stambulic T, Hassan SMA, Norman PA, Derry K, Payne DM, et al. Median sternotomy pain after cardiac surgery: To block, or not? A systematic review and meta-analysis. Journal of Cardiac Surgery. 2022;**37**(11):3729-3742

[56] Maeßen T, Korir N, Van de Velde M, Kennes J, Pogatzki-Zahn E, Joshi GP, et al. Pain management after cardiac surgery via median sternotomy: A systematic review with procedure-specific postoperative pain management (PROSPECT) recommendations. European Journal of Anaesthesiology. 1 Oct 2023;**40**(10):758-768

[57] Sepolvere G, Tognu A, Tedesco M, Coppolino F, Cristiano L. Avoiding the internal mammary artery during parasternal blocks: Ultrasound identification and technique considerations. Journal of Cardiothoracic and Vascular Anesthesia. 2021;**35**(6):1594-1602

[58] de la Torre PA, Garcia PD, Alvarez SL, Miguel FJ, Perez MF. A novel ultrasound-guided block: A promising alternative for breast analgesia. Aesthetic Surgery Journal. 2014;**34**(1):198-200

[59] McDonald SB, Jacobsohn E, Kopacz DJ, Desphande S, Helman JD, Salinas F, et al. Parasternal block and local anesthetic infiltration with levobupivacaine after cardiac surgery with desflurane: The effect on postoperative pain, pulmonary function, and tracheal extubation times. Anesthesia and Analgesia. 2005;**100**(1):25-32

[60] Pascarella G, Costa F, Nonnis G, Strumia A, Sarubbi D, Schiavoni L, et al. Ultrasound guided parasternal block for perioperative analgesia in cardiac surgery: A prospective study. Journal of Clinical Medicine. 6 Mar 2023;**12**(5):2060

[61] Kaya C, Dost B, Dokmeci O, Yucel SM, Karakaya D. Comparison of ultrasound-guided pecto-intercostal fascial block and Transversus thoracic muscle plane block for acute Poststernotomy pain management after cardiac surgery: A prospective, randomized, double-blind pilot study. Journal of Cardiothoracic and Vascular Anesthesia. 2022;**36**(8 PT A):2313-2321

[62] Sepolvere G, Fusco P, Tedesco M, Scimia P. Bilateral ultrasound-guided parasternal block for postoperative analgesia in cardiac surgery: Could it be the safest strategy? Regional Anesthesia and Pain Medicine. 2020;**45**(4):316-317

[63] El-Boghdadly K, Pawa A, Chin KJ. Local anesthetic systemic toxicity: Current perspectives. Local Regional Anesthesia. 2018;**11**:35-44

Chapter 6

Teaching Regional Anesthesia: Current Perspectives

Sandra Ximena Jaramillo-Rincón, Juliana María Galán Giraldo and María Alejandra Morales

Abstract

Regional anesthesia is an essential component of modern anesthesia practice, and there have been several changes in regional training methods in recent years. Effective anesthesia instructors must possess both clinical expertise and practical teaching skills. In order to ensure that future generations of anesthesia providers receive high-quality education and training, it is essential to train anesthesia instructors in the latest educational techniques and technical skills. This chapter aims to provide practical resources and tools for effectively training anesthesia providers in anesthesia programs. These may include simulation-based training models, online educational modules, peer-to-peer mentoring programs, hands-on workshops, and, finally, effective feedback.

Keywords: regional anesthesia, medical education, training, workplace-based assessment, entrustable professional activities

1. Introduction

The high demand for regional anesthesia in adults and children in the last 20 years has represented one of the most critical global changes in anesthesia [1–3]. The advantages, in medical quality and socioeconomic terms, are associated with the increased safety performance of the procedures and the routine usage of ultrasound techniques, increasing the success rate and reducing the number of complications and costs associated with perioperative care.

The success of the use of regional anesthesia techniques, however, is linked mostly to the experience of the operator, not only in the procedural sphere but also in clinical reasoning. It is essential to guarantee the anesthesiologist, both in training and in practice, a teaching-learning process based on deliberate practice and mastery learning that guarantees learning and continuous improvement of professional performance [4, 5].

Although the literature reports a significant gap in the confidence of anesthesia residents to perform regional anesthesia procedures without supervision, there needs to be more evidence about the best way to teach regional anesthesia skills [5, 6]. The anesthesiologists can consult the Guidelines for Training in Regional Anesthesia, published in 2005 and revised every 3 years by the American Society of Regional Anesthesia and Pain Medicine; these are the consensus guidelines regarding learning objectives and curricular content [7–9]. This chapter addresses the fundamental aspects of the teaching framework in complementary form, not only at the training level during residency programs but also in supra-specialized training programs and throughout life.

2. How to learn to do technical procedures?

A *practical or procedural skill* is defined as any mental and motor activity that requires the execution of a manual task, regardless of its degree of difficulty. Anesthesia professionals must undergo training to achieve competency in a range of skills to enable them to work safely in complex, dynamic, and unpredictable clinical environments. Acquiring competency in procedural skills therefore is an essential goal of anesthesia programs, with the expectation that a graduate should be proficient in basic procedural and clinical skills and ability to assume responsibility for safe patient care upon entry into the profession.

There are different and complementary approaches to understanding the teaching and learning of procedural skills. We recommend a practical model that combines the procedural skill taxonomy of Anita Harrow and Taylor et al.'s framework (**Figure 1**) [10].

The taxonomy devised by Anita Harrow provides a clear and definitive breakdown of the five essential stages that every anesthesia provider must master. These stages have a strong correlation with the Dreyfus and Dreyfus level of competence, as demonstrated in **Figure 1**. Moreover, Taylor et al. have presented a concrete six-stage educational framework for procedural skill training in medicine that emphasizes deliberate practice and domain enhancement. These six stages encompass Learning, Seeing, Practicing, Probing, and Maintaining, which are expertly adapted from the conventional four-stage Peyton model, as depicted in **Figure 1**.

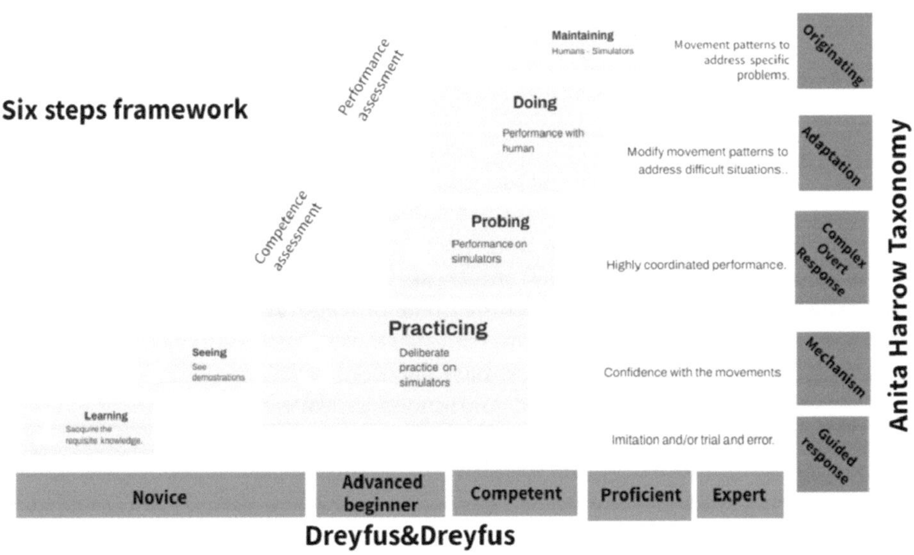

Figure 1.
Proposed pedagogical frameworks for procedural skills acquisition in medicine. Source: Adapted of Sawyer, T. et al. [10].

3. What skills do regional anesthesiologists need to learn and how to teach them?

Each practical skill that an anesthesiologist needs to learn (e.g., airway management, regional techniques, and invasive access) has a specific task. In the regional anesthesia skills case training, the students must learn different technical, cognitive, and behavioral skills (**Figure 2**) [3, 11].

3.1 Cognitive skills

Cognitive capabilities encompass a range of abilities that allow a person to comprehend, deduce, recall, organize, and transform data into fresh perspectives; make informed choices; tackle challenges; and gain knowledge. Within the domain of cognition, it is essential to have a thorough understanding of anatomy and sonoanatomy concepts and familiarity with equipment, medications, and anesthesia techniques [5, 12, 13]. Mastering these areas can significantly enhance cognitive abilities and facilitate optimal performance [14].

3.1.1 Teaching human anatomy for regional anesthesia

A comprehensive understanding of human anatomy, particularly nerve pathways and structures relevant to the specific region they will be targeting is necessary for the learning and proper execution of techniques in regional anesthesia. Accurately identifying nerves and optimizing block placement depend on this knowledge. Understanding the human body's structure and function is fundamental to regional anesthesia performance. Sonoanatomy, which involves using ultrasound to visualize anatomical structures in real time during medical procedures, is an essential skill in the field. A combination of didactic lectures, hands-on practical sessions, and interactive learning experiences is necessary to teach these skills effectively [1, 6, 7, 11–13, 15, 16].

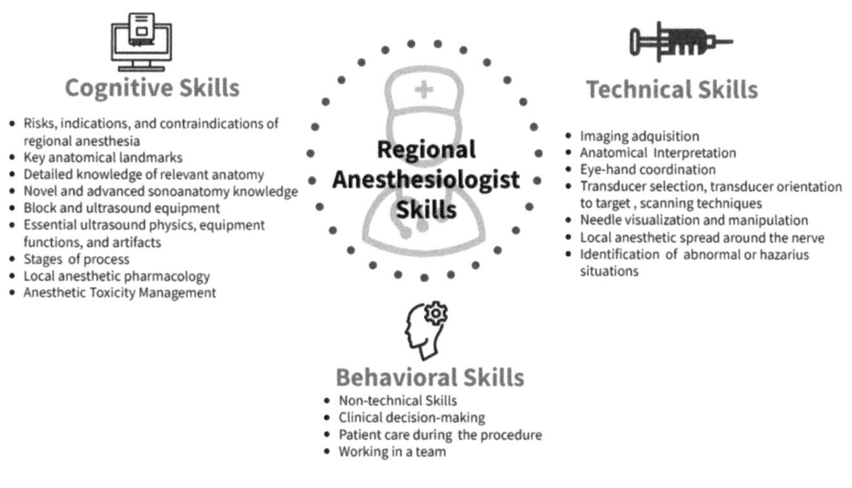

Figure 2.
Regional anesthesia skills.

Experienced instructors are crucial in guiding learners' progress and addressing individual challenges. By integrating diverse teaching strategies, medical educators can effectively equip students and practitioners with the necessary anatomical and sonoanatomical skills, ensuring their competency and success in clinical practice [5, 10, 14, 17].

3.1.1.1 Lectures

Lectures as a teaching strategy can be highly effective when supplemented with multiple practical activities that enable students to bridge the gap between theory and practice. A recent scoping review on effective teaching strategies in surface anatomy has highlighted the importance of adopting a multimodal approach [18, 19]. Literature shows great acceptance of small-group teaching by medical instructors, integrated clinical skills sessions, and incorporation of anatomical plastic models and cadaveric specimens in their anatomy classes [19, 20].

To further enrich the learning experience, several additional strategies can be implemented [18]. Clinical-applied teaching, for instance, can be introduced to provide students with real-life medical scenarios that demonstrate the practical application of anatomical knowledge. The use of radiological imaging can also prove beneficial in helping students visualize anatomical structures in a clinical context [3, 21]. Moreover, engaging activities like body painting and topographical body massage can make learning interactive and improve the student's performance [18].

By combining traditional lectures with these practical and engaging teaching methods, educators can create a dynamic and comprehensive learning environment that fosters a deeper understanding and appreciation of surface anatomy, contextualizes the teaching, embraces experiential learning, and facilitates the process [18, 22].

3.1.1.2 Videos, online modules, and virtual simulators

Explanatory videos and self-directed interactive virtual simulations are the most common and effective anatomy learning strategies. Research shows that virtual simulators can improve residents' skills by up to 40%. A specific study evaluated the impact of a short educational video with an interactive simulation on ultrasound anatomy knowledge. The results showed that the video significantly improved theoretical knowledge but, surprisingly, did not translate into an improvement in practical ultrasound scanning skills to locate the nerve. However, combining these strategies with supervised practical learning models can enhance student performance. For instance, a training module that included a didactic lecture on ultrasound-facilitated neuraxial anesthesia and mentored teaching on cadaveric spine dissections and hands-on ultrasound scanning of live models resulted in superior performance by the residents compared to those who only received the didactic lecture.

Woodworth et al. believed that exposition to an educational video of relevant anatomical structures plus simulation could improve the ability to interpret and recognize structures on ultrasound. They compared an experimental group that was exposed to the teaching video and 5 minutes of simulation and a control group that watched a comedy video without simulation. They had a written pretest and a posttest and an ultrasound scanning pre- and posttest in live models. They found that watching a video improved the knowledge of anatomy structures and image interpretation but could not demonstrate improvement in scanning nerves at hands-on practice [16].

They confirm that video and computer simulations are tools that can improve explicit knowledge, which in peripheral nerve blocks (PNB) is represented by the recognition of anatomic structures and their localization around the nerve, so this can make a difference against residents or fellows who do not have the opportunity to practice in simulation scenarios [16].

Access to an interactive ultrasound spine module improves theoretical knowledge and practical skills before clinical care. In summary, using explanatory videos and interactive simulations is valuable for learning, but when complemented with supervised practical experience, it significantly enhances the development of skills and knowledge.

3.1.1.3 Cadaver review sessions

Studies have shown that by including cadaver review sessions (CRSs) in anesthesiology, programs can significantly enhance residents' understanding of intricate anatomical structures involved in specific blockages, along with facilitating the honing of skills in ultrasound and needle use. In turn, this reduces the number of complications arising during clinical practice following peripheral nerve blocks.

In a recent study by Cale et al. [23] residents from the first and third years of anesthesiology programs took part in a 2-hour CRS once a month in a human anatomy laboratory. An anatomist and an anesthesiologist with training in regional anesthesia led the session, guiding the residents through critical anatomic structures and assisting them in integrating this knowledge to perform ultrasound-guided peripheral nerve blocks in the cadavers.

At the end of the study, the residents reported feeling more confident in recognizing anatomical structures on cadavers and using ultrasound. Most residents preferred CRS over online modules, with some noting that the practice on cadavers was relevant to their training and clinical practice. Overall, the experience helped the residents improve their performance in PNB and broaden their knowledge, making them better equipped to provide quality patient care.

3.2 Technical skills in regional anesthesia

It is important to note that more than explicit knowledge is needed; motor skills must also be developed. Unfortunately, teaching motor skills is often overlooked. Learning motor skills requires practicing and repeating procedures until the learning curve stabilizes; this is reached by overcoming several domains [10, 11, 16].

In the case of regional anesthesia, the evolution of skill is characterized by three stages [3, 11, 24]. The first one is *cognitive*, in which the residents get the concept of the skill. In this stage, residents behave timidly, inconsistently, and inaccurately; make many mistakes while doing the task; and need help interacting with the environment. The second stage is *associative*, where movements get more fluid, there are fewer mistakes, and residents can interact with the care team or patient. The last stage is *autonomous*, where movements are consistent, mistakes are rare, and residents can recognize them, solve unexpected situations, concentrate on other issues, and connect with the care team and patient.

Teaching strategies to train more confident, independent, and proficient anesthesiologists have been described as follows: To learn a new task, they should start by knowing the expected outcome and setting specific goals. They can prepare by reading, watching videos, or observing a mentor. Then, they can make a deconstruction of the task. This means breaking down the procedure into more straightforward steps. After that, temporally distributed simulation sessions are helpful to practice segmentation by performing steps sequentially until they can complete the task. Following the simulation, deliberate practice can be carried out with the guidance of a teacher, who assesses the learning level of the resident and, according to that, allows the resident to perform a procedure. When the tasks that residents are asked to do are in their zone of proximal development, skill development gets stimulated and reinforced [3, 11, 17].

Finally, feedback allows the residents to compare their previous concepts of the tasks with their actual performance and to receive information about how the teacher perceived it [25]. The teacher must give the residents a chance to share their sensations of the performance; then, it is necessary to make constructive criticism, identify the need for improvement, and highlight what the residents have done correctly. This feedback at the procedure's end helps the residents strengthen their knowledge [26, 27].

In this way, regional anesthesia trainers must master various needle insertion techniques with precision, including single or multiple injections. Utilizing ultrasound guidance is crucial for accurate needle placement and improving patient safety during the procedure. In this case, the anesthesiologist needs other specific skills to improve their performance in this technique. Additionally, nerve stimulation techniques are fundamental for nerve localization, aiding in identifying nerve responses and further enhancing the accuracy of the regional block [1, 3, 8, 12, 13, 28].

3.2.1 How to teach technical skills?

The didactic component of the technical skills training provides a theoretical understanding of anatomical structures and their clinical relevance, while practical sessions, such as cadaver dissections simulations and live model workshops, develop tactile familiarity with anatomical landmarks and build confidence in needle techniques. Ultrasound simulators and patient simulations enhance sonoanatomy skills by providing a risk-free environment for real-time image interpretation and probe manipulation.

3.2.1.1 Simulation-based practices

Simulation-based training is an approach that employs artificial devices to recreate various clinical scenarios that resemble real-world experiences, providing an enhanced learning opportunity [3, 17]. The procedures or situations utilized in the simulation can be pre-planned, standardized, and practiced repeatedly without posing any risk to the patient. Although simulation-based training has gained popularity and is now integrated into several undergraduate and postgraduate programs, there is still much to be discovered concerning its potential [4, 6, 29].

3.2.1.1.1 Advantages of simulation teaching based practices

The literature has shown that simulation-based training increases clinical knowledge and skill acquisition compared to non-simulation training and conventional teaching tools [21, 30]. It is significantly more efficient and cost-effective than other teaching methods for learning ultrasound-guided regional anesthesia, reducing the learning curve time and optimizing the trainees' training time [1, 21].

Simulation-based training is a superior alternative to traditional training methods in the medical field. This approach enables medical professionals to perfect procedures safely before applying them to real patients, resulting in improved outcomes and lower healthcare costs [6, 14, 21, 31, 32]. Not only does this create a safe learning space, but it also allows for immediate and accurate feedback, which is crucial for boosting confidence and competence [14, 33]. Feedback should be ongoing, reflective, and provided within a secure learning environment to ensure optimal results [1–3, 14, 30].

Additionally, simulation-based training focuses on improving and acquiring competencies rather than on volume-based training [29]. Finally, simulation has proven to be highly desirable in those programs, individuals, or training settings where it is infrequent or nonexistent [34].

3.2.1.1.2 Types of simulators on regional anesthesia

Among the variety of prototypes used in clinical simulation in regional anesthesia training are the following:

a. *Cadaveric sessions*

Cadaveric sessions hold a special place in the training process since they allow for a 3-dimensional representation and tactile feedback, requiring visuospatial reasoning to perform an appropriate needle positioning and, ultimately, an adequate PNB [35]. Practicing on cadavers brings the learning process closer to reality, unlike online modules in a 2-dimensional plane. Lin et al. performed similar sessions with regional and pain anesthesia fellows, finding a positive response [31, 36]. They believe that trainees can benefit from the high fidelity of cadavers to make multiple PNBs and enhance their sonographic orientation, which otherwise cannot be done in the operating room for several reasons [31, 36]. To avoid these issues, using a simulation space, or "block room," has been suggested to lead to a safe learning environment without stress or the risk of complications of PNB [31, 37, 38].
Improving technical skills is crucial to gain expertise in performing procedures. Woodworth et al. suggest that this can be achieved by using dynamic ultrasound images to help trainees understand unclear anatomy [39].

b. *Ultrasound-guided training of simulated participants*

The simulated participant, often referred to as an "SP," is an individual specially trained to portray a particular role or scenario in simulated environments, such as medical simulations, educational simulations, or communication exercises. The key characteristic of an SP is their ability to realistically replicate the characteristics, behaviors, and emotions of a specific person or patient, contributing to the authenticity and immersion of the simulated experience [29]. This resource is limited to teaching, learning, and reviewing ultrasound fundamentals and sonoanatomy, which are fundamental for developing an adequate and successful regional block technique [1]. It also improves the confidence and skill in using the ultrasound machine in invasive patients, reducing technique times and complications [6].

c. Ultrasound-guided training on manikins

There are exceptional ultrasound simulators on the market that provide realistic images and enable students to perform a wide range of procedures. These simulators are perfect for teaching basic skills such as identifying superficial anatomy and sonoanatomy and handling equipment and transducers [1, 30, 39]. They also offer training for more advanced skills, including needle handling, visualization, and the placement of local anesthetic or perineural catheters. However, it is important to note that these simulators come with high acquisition and maintenance costs and are not easily transportable.

d. Simulation crisis with manikins

This type of training is limited to management training in response to systemic toxicity of the local anesthetic. A disadvantage is that it prevents the trainee from assessing the possibilities of anatomical and pulse variants as anatomical repair in life patients [6].

e. Training on three-dimensional phantom models

This type of training improves understanding of anatomical principles and blocking techniques [6, 33]. It also enhances the novice trainees' needs focusing on anatomical principles and blocking techniques has improved novice trainees' needle orientation, hand-eye coordination, and understanding and recall of anatomy [32, 34]. These skills are crucial for the optimal development of a peripheral nerve block.
The 3D Phantom models used in ultrasound-guided regional anesthesia training are the Jelly Phantom, Meat Phantom, Elastomeric Rubber, and Cadaveric Piece. Each model has different processing dynamics but similar learning performances [21, 30, 32, 33]. Although some reports mention the high cost of using commercial models for this type of training, similar efficacy has been demonstrated in low-cost models [33].
Each model has different processing dynamics but similar learning performances (**Table 1**) [40]. Each one has different processing dynamics but similar learning performances, not to mention the trainer's perception of a more realistic environment with the cadaveric and meat models [1–3]. The literature requires more extensive descriptions of each simulation technique available today.

3.2.1.2 Clinical practice

Hands-on teaching in regional anesthesia involves a practical and experiential approach to training medical professionals in performing various nerve block techniques and procedures [13, 41]. In this educational method, learners actively engage in real-life situations, allowing them to gain firsthand experience and develop their skills in a supervised environment [23, 42]. By immersing themselves in the process, learners can better understand the intricacies of regional anesthesia, its challenges, and how to overcome them and allow the simulation phase [10, 11].

It is essential to recognize the value of hands-on teaching in regional anesthesia. This type of learning provides a dynamic experience that complements theoretical

Model used	Time for target identification	Time for task completion	Needle placement time	Characteristics
Transparent model	Shortest time	Shortest time	No significant difference	Less mistakes but less realistic
Opaque model	Longer time	Longer time	No significant difference	More realistic for learning target identification skills
Meat model	Longer time	Shortest time	No significant difference	Requires refrigeration, cannot be used after multiple needle uses, and is associated with more failures

Table 1.
Comparison of different low-cost models [33].

knowledge and helps learners bridge the gap between simulation and real-world practice [10]. By participating in hands-on training, medical professionals can refine their technical skills, improve decision-making, and enhance patient safety during regional anesthesia procedures. This interactive approach fosters a deeper understanding of the complexities and better prepares learners to handle real-life patient cases with greater competence and confidence [13, 43, 44].

Supervision is a critical aspect of hands-on teaching in regional anesthesia. Experienced mentors guide learners through the process, offering real-time feedback and constructive critiques [45, 46]. This close supervision ensures that learners perform procedures safely and effectively, minimizing the risk of complications and errors [28, 47]. Supervision may gradually decrease as learners progress, allowing them to develop their autonomy in regional anesthesia practice.

Gaining confidence and *autonomy* is a significant outcome of hands-on teaching in regional anesthesia [28]. As learners master different nerve block techniques and gain experience with various patient scenarios, they become more self-assured in their abilities [11, 48]. This newfound confidence empowers them to take on more complex cases and adapt their skills to different clinical situations [17]. Ultimately, hands-on teaching instills in learners a sense of autonomy, allowing them to provide high-quality regional anesthesia care independently and contribute positively to patient outcomes.

3.2.1.2.1 When is it suitable for a resident to conduct a regional block on a patient?

Defining the capability of a student to perform autonomous regional anesthesia involves assessing their proficiency, knowledge, and decision-making skills in executing these specialized tasks independently (see assessment session). Here are vital steps to determine a student's capability in autonomous regional blocks:

a. *Supervised Practice*: Allow the student to initially practice regional anesthesia techniques under direct supervision. Observe their performance, provide guidance, and assess their technical skills during this phase.

b. *Case Complexity*: Gradually expose the student to various complex cases. Evaluate their ability to choose appropriate regional anesthesia techniques based on patient needs, surgical requirements, and medical history.

c. *Patient Safety*: Assess the student's focus on patient safety throughout the process, including proper patient positioning, accurate nerve localization, and monitoring during the procedure.

d. *Decision-making:* Evaluate the student's ability to make critical decisions independently, such as choosing the appropriate nerve block technique, adjusting anesthesia dosage, and managing complications.

e. *Procedural Efficiency:* Assess the student's efficiency in performing regional anesthesia procedures, including time management and minimizing patient discomfort.

f. *Communication Skills:* Evaluate how effectively the student communicates with patients, colleagues, and other healthcare providers involved in the procedure.

g. *Documentation*: Review the student's ability to maintain accurate and comprehensive documentation of the regional anesthesia procedures, including preoperative assessments, procedural details, and postoperative care.

h. *Adherence to Guidelines*: Ensure the student follows established guidelines, protocols, and best practices for regional anesthesia, including infection control measures and patient consent procedures.

i. *Independent* Problem-solving: Observe how students handle unexpected challenges or complications during the procedure and assess their problem-solving skills.

j. *Self-assessment and Reflection*: Encourage the student to reflect on their performance, identify areas for improvement, and develop a plan for ongoing professional development.

k. *Gradual Autonomy:* Gradually allow the student to perform regional procedures with less direct supervision, increasing their level of autonomy as they demonstrate competence and confidence.

l. *Continuous Feedback:* Provide regular and constructive feedback to the students throughout the assessment process, helping them understand their strengths and areas for growth.

By following these steps and considering multiple aspects of the student's performance, educators can accurately determine the capability of the student to autonomously perform regional anesthesia procedures and confidently transition them to independent practice in this specialized field.

3.3 Behavioral skills in regional anesthesia

Behavioral skills or anesthetists' nontechnical skills (ANTS) refer to a set of cognitive and social skills and personal resources that enable safe and efficient task performance beyond the technical aspects of anesthesia administration [49–51]. These skills are essential for anesthetists to ensure patient safety, effective communication, and efficient teamwork during surgical procedures. ANTS encompass various competencies, including situational awareness, communication, decision-making, teamwork, leadership, and adaptability. Situational awareness involves perceiving and comprehending the surgical environment, anticipating potential challenges, and responding appropriately [52].

Teaching ANTS requires a comprehensive and structured approach to ensure anesthetists develop these critical skills effectively. In the clinical practice of anesthesiology, the acquisition of ANTS is highly important [52, 53]. However, despite efforts to evaluate and improve these skills [53–55], training strategies are still needed. To reinforce automatic behaviors when handling complex and stressful situations, it is recommended to draw from other specialties such as interactive workshops, simulation-based training, horror rooms, role-playing games, and analysis of adverse events [54, 55].

To engage anesthetists actively, it is recommended to organize interactive workshops and simulation-based training sessions [56–58]. These simulations allow them to practice ANTS in realistic scenarios, thereby fostering decision-making, communication, and teamwork in a controlled environment. Debriefing sessions are also crucial as they encourage self-reflection, identify areas for improvement, and reinforce positive behaviors. Encouraging senior anesthetists with strong ANTS to act as role models for junior colleagues can also be highly beneficial.

Utilizing video-based training modules can showcase examples of ANTS in action, demonstrating effective communication, teamwork, and situational awareness in various clinical scenarios [59–61]. Integrate the use of case-based learning into the training, permit anesthetists to analyze and discuss real-life cases that highlight the importance of ANTS. This approach allows for practical application and critical thinking.

ANTS training should be an ongoing process, with continual training and practice. Anesthetists should be encouraged to practice and reinforce these skills in their daily practice [11, 17]. Refresher courses or periodic workshops should be offered to reinforce learning. An environment where anesthetists feel comfortable discussing challenges and sharing experiences related to ANTS should also be created, encouraging open communication and learning from each other's experiences.

4. How to assess student performance in regional anesthesia?

Assessment in anesthesia has traditionally been focused on evaluating clinical practice, patient interaction, and critical situation analysis at the end of the learning process [49]. However, it is crucial to prioritize real-time, sequential, and progressive process assessment; personalized learning; and feedback throughout this process [62].

4.1 Entrustable professional activities (EPAs) and assessment

The emergence of Entrustable Professional Activities (EPAs) has led to a call for change in medical and health profession curricula. EPAs are units of clinical practice, tasks, or responsibilities that students can perform without supervision once they have achieved the desired competency [28, 63–65]. Each EPA incorporates domains and subdomains of general competencies, integrated with specific content from the curriculum's educational programs. Didactic activities are designed from concrete daily experiences in clinical practice at different levels depending on the year of study [28, 64, 65]. Three strategies, namely, situated learning, deliberate practice, and reflection, are used to help students achieve reliable clinical activities [66].

EPAs and the Dreyfus and Dreyfus model are complementary frameworks that can assess and guide regional learners' progress and development. By aligning with competency-based medical education (CBME) principles, EPAs focus on learners' achievement of specific competencies instead of relying solely on time-based training. EPAs are measurable milestones that demonstrate a trainee's ability to conduct critical professional activities under appropriate supervision [67, 68]. The Dreyfus and Dreyfus model describes the stages of skill acquisition and expertise development, proposing five stages: Novice, Advanced Beginner, Competent, Proficient, and Expert. According to this model, individuals progress through these stages as they gain experience and expertise in a particular domain [10, 67, 68].

EPAs and the Dreyfus and Dreyfus model complement each other in medical education. EPAs can be mapped to the different stages of the Dreyfus and Dreyfus model. For instance, basic clinical skills required by EPAs might align with the Novice, Advanced, and Beginner stages. In contrast, complex decision-making and management may align with the Competent and Proficient stages [67, 68]. EPAs provide a concrete way to assess learners' abilities to perform specific professional activities. As learners progress through their training, they can be evaluated against EPAs, and their performance can be compared to the expectations associated with the corresponding Dreyfus and Dreyfus stages. This assessment process enables educators to provide targeted feedback and support for learners at different skill levels [69].

The Dreyfus and Dreyfus model underscores the gradual development of expertise and autonomy. EPAs can serve as markers of a learner's readiness to take on more responsibility and independence in their clinical practice as they transition from being supervised to being entrusted with certain professional activities [10, 11].

4.2 EPAS in regional anesthesia

The field of regional anesthesiology and acute pain medicine has recognized the need for standardizing assessments to effectively track trainee competency. The Accreditation Council for Graduate Medical Education (ACGME) provides competency descriptions and milestones, but other methods are necessary for accurate assessment [70]. To address this need, EPAs and special assessments models have emerged as promising approaches to evaluate the level of competency of residents and fellows.

To develop a comprehensive assessment framework, an expert group with experience in anesthesia education and competency assessment, established a list of 23 EPAs, a clearly defined entrustment scale, and a mapping to ACGME milestones [28]. This provides a standardized approach to assessing competency and ensuring well-prepared and competent fellows (**Table 2**). This rigorous methodology ensures that the RAAPM EPAs and procedural skills accurately reflect the required competencies for fellows, facilitating meaningful performance feedback.

EPA category	EPA title (assigned number)
Preoperative assessment	• Peripheral nerve block—regional procedure evaluation and informed consent (1) • Neuraxial technique—regional procedure evaluation and informed consent • Preoperative assessment of the patient with preexisting neurological dysfunction for regional anesthesia • Preoperative assessment of the patient on altered coagulation for regional anesthesia • Evaluation and management of a patient with postoperative pain requiring rescue analgesia in the PACU
Patients with special conditions	• Evaluation and management of regional anesthesia in the geriatric patient • Evaluation and management of a patient with complex pain history • Evaluation and management of regional anesthesia in a trauma patient • Evaluation and management of acute pain in a pediatric patient
Perioperative care	• Evaluation and management of a patient that would benefit from regional anesthesia of the upper extremity. • Evaluation and management of a patient that would benefit from regional anesthesia of the lower extremity. • Evaluation for and placement of a continuous peripheral nerve block • Evaluation and management of a patient that would benefit from regional anesthesia of the thorax. • Evaluation and management of a patient that would benefit from regional anesthesia of the abdomen. • Perioperative management of a neuraxial block for surgical anesthesia • Perioperative management of a peripheral or truncal nerve block for surgical anesthesia • Appropriate conduct of handoff/transfer of care with an emphasis on minimizing barriers to communication
Regional and acute pain service	• Postoperative evaluation and management of patients with continuous peripheral nerve blocks. • Postoperative evaluation and management of patients with continuous neuraxial catheters (19). Postoperative evaluation and management of the ambulatory patient with a continuous peripheral nerve block. • Management of an inpatient acute pain service. Evaluation and management of acute pain in the nonoperative setting
Other	Recognition, evaluation, and management of complications or potential complications related to regional anesthesia and acute pain management including assessment, documentation, and disclosure.

Table 2.
List of entrustable professional activities (EPAs) [28].

4.3 Regional anesthesia and clinical competence

Assessing trainees' proficiency in regional anesthesia aligns well with Miller's Pyramid of Clinical Competence. At the pyramid's base lies "Knows," where learners acquire factual knowledge about regional anesthesia techniques, relevant anatomy, and pharmacology. Moving up, "Knows How" reflects their ability to demonstrate the procedural steps and principles in controlled environments, such as simulation

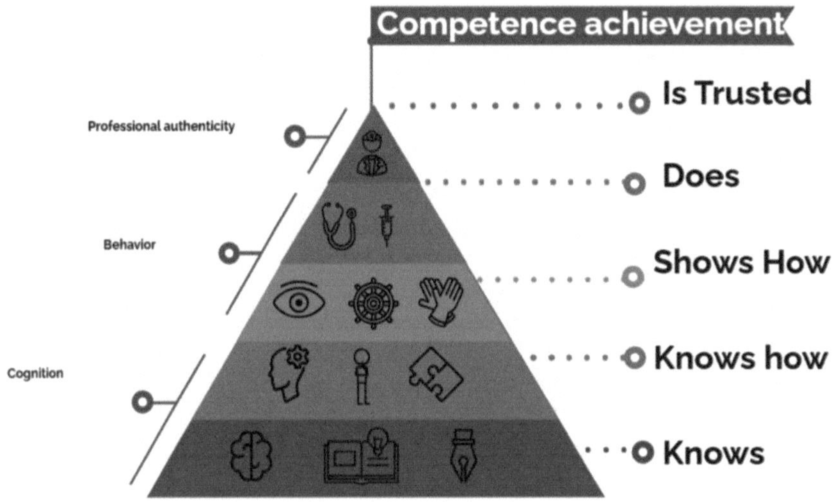

Figure 3.
Extending Miller's pyramid. Source: Adapted of Ten Cate et al. [67].

labs. The next level, "Shows How," pertains to their ability to apply regional anesthesia under direct supervision in natural clinical settings. The final and more recent level "Is Trusted" included by Ten Cate et al. (**Figure 3**) [67].

As trainees gain experience and competence, they also progress to higher levels of Miller's Pyramid. "Does," the penultimate level, signifies the point at which trainees can perform regional anesthesia more autonomously, though with some guidance and oversight. Finally, the pyramid's pinnacle is "Does Independently," where learners exhibit mastery in regional anesthesia and can administer it safely and effectively without supervision [62, 67].

Overall, the assessment of EPAs like regional anesthesia aligns with the progression of competence achievement at Miller's Pyramid, ensuring that trainees advance through stages of knowledge and competence, ultimately becoming skilled and independent practitioners in anesthesiology. This structured approach to assessment enhances patient safety and ensures a high standard of care in clinical practice.

Evaluating the skill level of trainees in regional anesthesia follows the framework of Miller's Pyramid of Clinical Competence. The pyramid's base is "Knows," where learners acquire knowledge of regional anesthesia techniques, relevant anatomy, and pharmacology. Moving up, "Knows How" reflects their ability to demonstrate procedural steps and principles in controlled environments, like simulation labs. The next level, "Shows How," pertains to their ability to apply regional anesthesia under direct supervision in natural clinical settings.

When trainees reach "Does", they achieve the second-to-last level. This one signifies the point at which trainees can perform regional anesthesia more independently but with some guidance and supervision. Finally, the pyramid's peak is "Does Independently," where learners demonstrate mastery in regional anesthesia and can administer it safely and effectively without supervision.

Overall, the assessment of Entrustable Professional Activities (EPAs) such as regional anesthesia aligns with the progression of competence achievement at Miller's Pyramid. This approach ensures that trainees advance through stages of knowledge and competence, ultimately becoming skilled and independent practitioners in

Test	Reliability	Validity	Feasibility	Educational impact	Assessment target
Procedure logs	Low self-reporting, there may be errors and omissions	Low, there is no guarantee that the procedure will be carried out properly	Easy	Low	Technical skills
Procedure logs with a minimum number	Low self-reporting, there may be errors and omissions	Low, there is no guarantee that the procedure will be carried out properly	Easy to use	Low	Technical skills
Direct unstructured observation	Low	High apparent validity	Easy to use	Potentially high	Technical, nontechnical skills
Checklists and global rating scales (OSAT)	Good for observers trained in the educational context	High construct validity in epidural punctures, interscalene block	Easy to use, but requires training	High, depending on context	Technical, nontechnical skills
Naik scale	High	High	High	High, correlation with expertise level	Technical skills
Regional anesthesia procedural skills (RAPS) tool	High	High internal and external validity	Applicable to any type of block; using ultrasound or without surface anatomy-based techniques	High correlation with expertise level	Technical skills
McLeod checklist	High	High internal validity	Easy to use	High correlation with expertise level	Technical skills
Objective assessment tool (OAT)	High	High internal validity	Easy to use	High correlation with expertise level in clinical setting	Technical skills
Direct Observation of Procedural Skills (DOPS)	Good for observers trained in the educational context	Constructive validity in epidural punctures, interscalene block	Easy to use, but requires training	High, depending on context	Technical skills
Feedback 360	Moderate for non-trained observers	High	Expensive, time-consuming	Very High	Technical, nontechnical skills
Simulation-based assessment	Depends on the assessment instrument and regional model	Apparent validity, highly variable in any context	High cost related to the type of simulation used	Depends on the selected assessment tool	Technical, nontechnical skills
Objective Structured Assessment of Technical Skills (OSAT)	Good for observers trained in the educational context	High in ultrasound-guided regional anesthesia	Expensive, time-consuming, and requires special installations	Potentially high	Technical skills

Test	Reliability	Validity	Feasibility	Educational impact	Assessment target
Video-feedback	Excellent	Technical and nontechnical skills	Time-consuming and requires special equipment	High	Technical, nontechnical skills
Gaze pattern analysis	High	High, non-observer-dependent	High cost, requires special equipment	Moderate	Technical, nontechnical skills
Imperial College Surgical Assessment Device (ICSAD)	High	High, non-observer-dependent	High cost, requires previous training	Moderate	Technical skills
Anesthesia-Clinical Evaluation Exercise (A-CEX)	High	High	Easy, needs training to use	High	Technical, nontechnical skills

Table 3.
Assessment tools used in regional anesthesia [49, 73].

anesthesiology. This structured methodology enhances patient safety and guarantees a high standard of care in clinical practice.

4.4 Assessment tools for regional anesthesia

In the field of regional anesthesia, programmatic assessment is utilized to evaluate the progress and competence of learners in a systematic and comprehensive manner [71]. This approach differs from traditional assessment methods that rely on individual examinations, as programmatic assessment involves continuous and longitudinal data collection through various tools and activities. These may include direct observations, simulation-based assessments, case-based discussions, and feedback from both faculty and patients. By gathering data over time, program directors and educators can gain a holistic view of the trainees' abilities, identifying strengths and areas for improvement. This approach fosters a culture of continuous learning and improvement, allowing for tailored interventions and support to enhance the learners' proficiency in regional anesthesia [49, 72, 73]. Moreover, programmatic assessment provides a more accurate and reliable representation of a trainee's overall competency, ensuring that they are well-prepared to deliver safe and effective regional anesthesia services upon completing their training.

To enhance the effectiveness of programmatic assessment, various assessment tools have been proven helpful in the van der Vleuten assessment equation (**Table 3**).

4.5 Feedback as assessment tool

Receiving feedback is essential for improving the learning process when acquiring, practicing, and reflecting on clinical skills [25]. However, trainers and teachers may not be familiar with this pedagogical tool, which limits the execution of the feedback process. To provide optimal feedback when teaching regional anesthesia, follow these short and precise tips:

a. Wait for the student to request feedback.

b. Provide feedback in a timely manner when it is relevant.

c. Balance positive and negative actions in the feedback.

d. Conduct feedback in a safe and private environment, with mutual respect and an appropriate tone of voice.

e. Offer a clear improvement plan and encourage the learner to develop specific actions for growth.

f. Keep the feedback concise and avoid unnecessary information.

However, some barriers can hinder effective feedback, such as inadequate communication skills, making moral and personal judgments, defensive learners, and closed-mindedness. By following these guidelines and being mindful of potential barriers, teachers and learners can ensure a more productive feedback process when teaching regional anesthesia.

5. Conclusions

In conclusion, anesthesiologists must be able to perform regional anesthesia with expertise and diminishing risks for the patients. To achieve that, anesthesiology programs should combine theoretical knowledge and strategical teaching to develop motor skills. Thus, it is imperative to have high-quality training before trainees or residents face actual patients. This training can involve multiple strategies such as lectures, multimedia, cadaver review sessions, simulation-based practices with manikins and ultrasound, and hands-on and supervised clinical practice and deliberate practice. This chapter allows to understand the way trainees learn and provides some useful tools that can be used to implement accurate procedural skills teaching and learning techniques, leading to more confident anesthesiologists and better results at performing regional anesthesia [74–76].

Acknowledgements

The authors thank Ernesto Rojas MD, Alexandra Vargas MD, German Gutierrez MD, and Juliana Salazar MD for taking part of their time to read this chapter and contribute to the final product.

Conflict of interest

The authors declare no conflict of interest.

Abbreviations

ANTS	anesthetists' nontechnical skills
CBME	competency-based medical education
CRS	cadaver review sessions
DOPS	direct observation of procedural skills
EPAs	entrustable professional activities (EPAs)
ICSAD	Imperial College surgical assessment device
OAT	objective assessment tool
OSAT	objective structured assessment of technical skills
PNB	peripheral nerve blocks
RAPS	regional anesthesia procedural skills
SP	simulated participant
US	ultrasound

Author details

Sandra Ximena Jaramillo-Rincón[1,2]*, Juliana María Galán Giraldo[1] and María Alejandra Morales[1]

1 Universidad de Los Andes, Bogotá, Colombia

2 Clinica de Marly, Bogotá, Colombia

*Address all correspondence to: sx.jaramillo@uniandes.edu.co

References

[1] Nix CM et al. A scoping review of the evidence for teaching ultrasound-guided regional anesthesia. Regional Anesthesia and Pain Medicine. 2013;**38**(6):471-480

[2] Cozowicz C, Poeran J, Memtsoudis SG. Epidemiology, trends, and disparities in regional anaesthesia for orthopaedic surgery. British Journal of Anaesthesia. 2015;**115**(Suppl. 2):ii57-ii67

[3] Kim TE, Tsui BCH. Simulation-based ultrasound-guided regional anesthesia curriculum for anesthesiology residents. Korean Journal of Anesthesiology. 2019;**72**(1):13-23

[4] Asaad BO et al. A survey on teaching ultrasound-guided chronic pain procedures in pain medicine fellowship programs. Pain Physician. 2014;**17**(6):E681-E689

[5] Chelly JE et al. Training of residents in peripheral nerve blocks during anesthesiology residency. Journal of Clinical Anesthesia. 2002;**14**(8):584-588

[6] Broking K, Waurick R. How to teach regional anesthesia. Current Opinion in Anaesthesiology. 2006;**19**(5):526-530

[7] Hargett MJ et al. Guidelines for regional anesthesia fellowship training. Regional Anesthesia and Pain Medicine. 2005;**30**(3):218-225

[8] Regional A. Acute pain medicine fellowship directors, guidelines for fellowship training in regional anesthesiology and acute pain medicine: Third edition, 2014. Regional Anesthesia and Pain Medicine. 2015;**40**(3):213-217

[9] Regional A. Acute pain medicine fellowship directors, guidelines for fellowship training in regional anesthesiology and acute pain medicine: Second edition, 2010. Regional Anesthesia and Pain Medicine. 2011;**36**(3):282-288

[10] Sawyer T et al. Learn, see, practice, prove, do, maintain: An evidence-based pedagogical framework for procedural skill training in medicine. Academic Medicine. 2015;**90**(8):1025-1033

[11] Slater RJ, Castanelli DJ, Barrington MJ. Learning and teaching motor skills in regional anesthesia: A different perspective. Regional Anesthesia and Pain Medicine. 2014;**39**(3):230-239

[12] Chuan A et al. Non-fellowship regional anesthesia training and assessment: An international Delphi study on a consensus curriculum. Regional Anesthesia and Pain Medicine. 2021;**46**(10):867-873

[13] Haskins SC et al. American Society of Regional Anesthesia and Pain Medicine expert panel recommendations on point-of-care ultrasound education and training for regional anesthesiologists and pain physicians-part I: Clinical indications. Regional Anesthesia and Pain Medicine. 2021;**46**(12):1031-1047

[14] Burgess A et al. Tips for teaching procedural skills. BMC Medical Education. 2020;**20**(Suppl. 2):458

[15] Neal JM et al. Regional anesthesia and pain medicine: US Anesthesiology resident training-the year 2015. Regional Anesthesia and Pain Medicine. 2017;**42**(4):437-441

[16] VanderWielen BA et al. Teaching sonoanatomy to anesthesia faculty and residents: Utility of hands-on gel

phantom and instructional video training models. Journal of Clinical Anesthesia. 2015;**27**(3):188-194

[17] Lee Wiggins L et al. Using evidence-based best practices of simulation, checklists, deliberate practice, and debriefing to develop and improve a regional anesthesia training course. AANA Journal. 2018;**86**(2):119-126

[18] Abu Bakar YI et al. A scoping review of effective teaching strategies in surface anatomy. Anatomical Sciences Education. 2022;**15**(1):166-177

[19] Louw G, Eizenberg N, Carmichael SW. The place of anatomy in medical education: AMEE guide no 41. Medical Teacher. 2009;**31**(5):373-386

[20] Edmunds S, Brown G. Effective small group learning: AMEE guide No. 48. Medical Teacher. 2010;**32**(9):715-726

[21] Chen XX et al. Ultrasound-guided regional anesthesia simulation training: A systematic review. Regional Anesthesia and Pain Medicine. 2017;**42**(6):741-750

[22] Johnson EO, Charchanti AV, Troupis TG. Modernization of an anatomy class: From conceptualization to implementation. A case for integrated multimodal-multidisciplinary teaching. Anesthesia Science Education. 2012;**5**(6):354-366

[23] Vanka A, Hovaguimian A. Teaching strategies for the clinical environment. The Clinical Teacher. 2019;**16**(6):570-574

[24] Sewell JL et al. Trainee perception of cognitive load during observed faculty staff teaching of procedural skills. Medical Education. 2019;**53**(9):925-940

[25] Bosse HM et al. The benefit of repetitive skills training and frequency of expert feedback in the early acquisition of procedural skills. BMC Medical Education. 2015;**15**:22

[26] Udani AD et al. Comparative-effectiveness of simulation-based deliberate practice versus self-guided practice on resident anesthesiologists' acquisition of ultrasound-guided regional anesthesia skills. Regional Anesthesia and Pain Medicine. 2016;**41**(2):151-157

[27] Kilicaslan A et al. A simple, feedback-based simulation model for ultrasound-guided regional anaesthesia. Indian Journal of Anaesthesia. 2012;**56**(4):431-433

[28] Porter S, Prendiville E, Allen BFS et al. Development of entrustable professional activities for regional anesthesia and pain medicine fellowship training. Regional Anesthesia and Pain Medicine. 2022;**47**:672-677

[29] Nestel D et al. Values and value in simulated participant methodology: A global perspective on contemporary practices. Medical Teacher. 2018;**40**(7):697-702

[30] Li J, Szabova A. Ultrasound-guided nerve blocks in the head and neck for chronic pain management: The anatomy, sonoanatomy, and procedure. Pain Physician. 2021;**24**(8):533-548

[31] Cale AS et al. Integrating a cadaver review session into the existing regional anesthesia training for anesthesiology residents: An initial experience. Medical Science Educator. 2020;**30**(2):695-703

[32] Kessler J et al. Teaching concepts in ultrasound-guided regional anesthesia. Current Opinion in Anaesthesiology. 2016;**29**(5):608-613

[33] Liu Y et al. Comparison of the development of performance skills in ultrasound-guided regional anesthesia simulations with different phantom models. Simulation in Healthcare. 2013;**8**(6):368-375

[34] Novak-Jankovic V. Simulation-based training of regional anesthesia medical simulation center, university medical center Ljubljana, Slovenia. Acta Clinica Croatica. 2022;**61**(Suppl. 2):155-159

[35] Kessler J, Moriggl B, Grau T. Ultrasound-guided regional anesthesia: Learning with an optimized cadaver model. Surgical and Radiologic Anatomy. 2014;**36**(4):383-392

[36] Lin DC et al. Letter to the editor on: "Integrating a cadaver review session into the existing regional anesthesia training for anesthesiology residents: An initial experience". Medical Science Educator. 2022;**32**(3):755

[37] Sehmbi H, Johnson M, Dhir S. Ultrasound-guided subomohyoid suprascapular nerve block and phrenic nerve involvement: A cadaveric dye study. Regional Anesthesia and Pain Medicine. 2019;**44**(5):561-564

[38] Maikong N et al. Cadaveric study investigating the phrenic-sparing volume for anterior suprascapular nerve block. Regional Anesthesia and Pain Medicine. 2021;**46**(9):769-772

[39] Woodworth GE et al. Efficacy of computer-based video and simulation in ultrasound-guided regional anesthesia training. Journal of Clinical Anesthesia. 2014;**26**(3):212-221

[40] Hocking G, Hebard S, Mitchell CH. A review of the benefits and pitfalls of phantoms in ultrasound-guided regional anesthesia. Regional Anesthesia and Pain Medicine. 2011;**36**(2):162-170

[41] Kim TE et al. Implementation of clinical practice changes by experienced anesthesiologists after simulation-based ultrasound-guided regional anesthesia training. Korean Journal of Anesthesiology. 2017;**70**(3):318-326

[42] Ramani S, Leinster S. AMEE guide no. 34: Teaching in the clinical environment. Medical Teacher. 2008;**30**(4):347-364

[43] Souzdalnitski D, Narouze S. Clinical expertise in regional anesthesia: Anesthesiologists voice their need for formal training. Saudi Journal of Anaesthesia. 2013;**7**(4):371-372

[44] Cooper AZ, Simpson D, Nordquist J. Optimizing the physical clinical learning environment for teaching. Journal of Graduate Medical Education. 2020;**12**(2):221-222

[45] Kilminster SM, Jolly BC. Effective supervision in clinical practice settings: A literature review. Medical Education. 2000;**34**(10):827-840

[46] Sato H, Yukawa K, Doi M. Supervision of new surgical procedures in Japan: Current practice and supervision issues at university hospitals in Japan. Surgery. 2020;**168**(6): 1109-1114

[47] Feeley AA et al. Evaluating the impact of supervision on surgical trainees stress response during simulated surgical procedures; a crossover randomized trial. Journal of Surgical Education. 2022;**79**(6):1379-1386

[48] de Oliveira Filho GR, Mettrau FAC. The effect of high-frequency, structured expert feedback on the learning curves of basic interventional ultrasound skills applied to regional anesthesia. Anesthesia and Analgesia. 2018;**126**(3):1028-1034

[49] Jaramillo-Rincón SX et al. Anesthesia assessment in the era of competences: State of the art. Colombian Journal of Anesthesiology. 2020;**48**(3):145-154

[50] Patey R, et al. Developing a taxonomy of Anesthetists' nontechnical skills (ANTS). In: Henriksen K, Battles JB, Marks ES, Lewin DI, editors. Advances in Patient Safety: From Research to Implementation (Volume 4: Programs, Tools, and Products). Rockville (MD): Agency for Healthcare Research and Quality (US); 2005 Feb. PMID: 21250033

[51] Flin R, Patey R. Non-technical skills for anaesthetists: Developing and applying ANTS. Best Practice & Research. Clinical Anaesthesiology. 2011;**25**(2):215-227

[52] Fletcher G et al. Anaesthetists' non-technical skills (ANTS): Evaluation of a behavioural marker system. British Journal of Anaesthesia. 2003;**90**(5):580-588

[53] Boet S et al. Measuring non-technical skills of anaesthesiologists in the operating room: A systematic review of assessment tools and their measurement properties. British Journal of Anaesthesia. 2018;**121**(6):1218-1226

[54] Youngson GG. Teaching and assessing non-technical skills. The Surgeon. 2011;**9**(Suppl. 1):S35-S37

[55] DeTata C. Teaching and assessing non-technical skills. The Clinical Teacher. 2015;**12**(3):219

[56] Peddle M. Participant perceptions of virtual simulation to develop non-technical skills in health professionals. Journal of Research in Nursing. 2019;**24**(3-4):167-180

[57] Mossenson AI et al. Promoting anaesthetisia providers' non-technical skills through the vital anaesthesia simulation training (VAST) course in a low-resource setting. British Journal of Anaesthesia. 2020;**124**(2):206-213

[58] Walsh CM et al. Non-technical skills curriculum incorporating simulation-based training improves performance in colonoscopy among novice endoscopists: Randomized controlled trial. Digestive Endoscopy. 2020;**32**(6):940-948

[59] Nagaraj MB et al. Using trauma video review to assess EMS handoff and trauma team non-technical skills. Prehospital Emergency Care. 2023;**27**(1):10-17

[60] Spanager L et al. Reliable assessment of general surgeons' non-technical skills based on video-recordings of patient simulated scenarios. American Journal of Surgery. 2013;**206**(5):810-817

[61] van Maarseveen OEC et al. Reliability of the assessment of non-technical skills by using video-recorded trauma resuscitations. European Journal of Trauma and Emergency Surgery. 2022;**48**(1):441-447

[62] Tetzlaff JE. Assessment of competency in anesthesiology. Anesthesiology. 2007;**106**(4):812-825

[63] Dabbagh A et al. The role of entrustable professional activities (EPAs) in competency-based medical education for anesthesiology residents: A pilot phase. Anesthesiology and Pain Medicine. 2022;**12**(5):e130176

[64] Woodworth GE et al. Development and pilot testing of entrustable professional activities (EPAs) for US anesthesiology residency training. Anesthesia and Analgesia. 2021;**132**(6):1579-1591

[65] Ganzhorn A et al. National consensus on Entrustable Professional

Activities (EPAs) for competency-based training in anaesthesiology. PLoS One. 2023;**18**(7):e0288197

[66] Ten Cate O. Nuts and bolts of Entrustable Professional Activities (EPAs). Journal of Graduate Medical Education. 2013;**5**(1):157-158

[67] Ten Cate O et al. Entrustment decision making: Extending Miller's pyramid. Academic Medicine. 2021;**96**(2):199-204

[68] Ten Cate O, Schumacher DJ. Professional Activities (EPAs) versus competencies and skills: Exploring why different concepts are often conflated. Advances in Health Sciences Education: Theory and Practice. 2022;**27**(2):491-499

[69] Peters H et al. Twelve tips for the implementation of EPAs for assessment and entrustment decisions. Medical Teacher. 2017;**39**(8):802-807

[70] Ambardekar A et al. Anesthesiology Milestones. [Internet]. The Accreditation Council for Graduate Medical Education. 2021. Available from: https://www.acgme.org/globalassets/pdfs/milestones/anesthesiologymilestones.pdf [Accessed: November 28, 2023]

[71] van der Vleuten CP et al. A model for programmatic assessment fit for purpose. Medical Teacher. 2012;**34**(3):205-214

[72] Beutler Crawford GL, Johnson B, Evans H. Assessment tools for the evaluation of simulation-based competency In ultrasound-guided regional anesthesia: An integrative review. AANA Journal. 2023;**91**(2):109-116

[73] Bamber H. Evaluation of the workplace-based assessment anaesthesia-clinical evaluation exercise (A-CEX) and its role in the Royal College of anaesthetists 2021 curriculum. Cureus. 2023;**15**(4):e37402

[74] Jačisko J, Mezian K, Güvener O, Ricci V, Kobesová A, Özçakar L. Mnemonics and metaphorical videos for teaching/learning musculoskeletal sonoanatomy. American Journal of Physical Medicine and Rehabilation. 2022;**101**(12):E189-E193

[75] People E. ESRA Europe [Internet]. ESRA. 2015. Available from: https://esraeurope.org/ [Accessed: July 29, 2023]

[76] NYSORA. World Leader in Anesthesiology Education [Internet]. NYSORA. 2022. Available from: https://www.nysora.com/ [Accessed: July 29, 2023]